Communication Skills
for Nurses

A practical guide on how to achieve successful consultations

Communication Skills for Nurses

A practical guide on how to achieve successful consultations

by Marilyn Edwards

QUAY
BOOKS

A division of MA Healthcare Ltd

Quay Books Division, MA Healthcare Ltd, St Jude's Church, Dulwich Road, London
SE24 0PB

British Library Cataloguing-in-Publication Data
A catalogue record is available for this book

© MA Healthcare Limited 2010
ISBN-10: 1 85642 393 X; ISBN-13: 978 1 85642 393 9

Printed by CLE, Huntingdon, Cambridgeshire

Contents

Acknowledgements

I would like to thank all my colleagues and friends who have offered constructive comments on specialist areas in the text. Special thanks to Heidi Cross and Sue Gribble, Paul Bowman, Michelle Price, Alison Troke and her colleagues, Marie Murphy and 'Ann'.

My husband Chris has supported me during my many hours of research and writing and his proof reading and comments from a lay perspective have been invaluable.

Preface

Over a third of all consultations in general practice are conducted by nurses, having risen from 27% in 1995 to 35% in 2007 (Hippisley-Cox and Jumbu, 2008). This coincides with the increase of practice nurse numbers from 10 082 in 1997 to 14 554 in 2007 (The NHS Information Centre, 2008).

Chambers (2008) provides definitions for consultation and skill thus:

Consultation - a deliberation, or a meeting for deliberation.

Skill - expertness, aptitudes and competencies appropriative for a particular job, expert knowledge.

Consultation skills for practice nurses can be described as the competencies and expertise to interact with patients in a deliberative manner.

The consultation is the key element of primary care as patients are more satisfied with the care given by clinicians who have demonstrated good communication skills. Poor communication or dissatisfaction with a consultation is reported to be a major reason why patients decide not to attend appointments, or do not take prescribed treatment (Miles, 2008). Patients need to be satisfied with the consultation, understand their condition, and understand the reasons for their treatment or management plan.

Over a third of all consultations are no longer soley the domain of medical practitioners as nurses increasingly become the first contact for patients (Kaufman, 2008). Nurses consult with patients during every interaction, from arranging an appointment on the telephone, throughout the consultation, or during follow up contact. Good consultation skills have always been relevant to nurses but as the role develops it is essential that these skills continue to improve. Patients are reported to value the care and support given by nurses who offered more advice on self-care and management than doctors (Baird, 2006).

This book has been written to reinforce good consultation skills and highlight areas where individual readers might wish to review and improve their own consultation techniques, through case histories and scenarios that are likely to be common in many practices. Although the text and scenarios relate to practice nurse consultations, the content can be transferred to all primary care nursing settings. It is acknowledged that nurses can be male or female, but for simplicity in the text, the nurse is referred to as female.

Baird A (2006) The Consultation. *Nurse Prescriber.* **9**(3). www.nurse-prescriber.co.uk accessed 29/3/2009

Chambers (2008) *The Chambers Dictionary* 11th Ed. Edinburgh, Chambers Harrap Publishers Ltd

Hippisley-Cox J & Jumbu G (2008) *Trends in Consultation Rates in General Practice 1995-2007: Analysis of the QRESEARCH database.* London, The NHS Information Centre

Kaufman G (2008) Patient assessment: effective consultation and history taking. *Nursing Standard.* **23**(4): 50-6

Miles J (2008) Effective communication. *Practice Nurse.* **35**(2): 42-7

The NHS Information Centre (2008) *General and Personal Medical Services England 1997-2007.* London, The NHS Information Centre

Introduction

"Patients in their journey through the health care system are entitled to be treated with respect and honesty, and to be involved wherever possible in decisions about their treatment."

(Kennedy, 2001)

Improving the patients' experience of health care is the central purpose of clinical governance. Patients have given consistent feedback about what matters to them (Department of Health, 2003). Good care means:
- Getting good treatment – high quality, safe and effective treatment delivered by capable teams.
- Being safe and comfortable – confidence in the care environment.
- Being informed and having a say in the care they receive.
- Being treated as a person – with respect, honesty and dignit (Royal College of Nursing, 2008).

These issues should be present at every point of contact with health services. The journey includes health awareness, access to care, continuity of care and support for carers. But people may face additional challenges. For example, people whose first language is not English may have problems with information and accessing care. The management of equity, diversity and choice also influence the patient experience.

A lack of attention to the pre-consultation period can adversely affect clinical reasoning, perceptual skills and the ability to perform effectively and impartially in the consultation (Chafer 2003, cited by Kaufman, 2008). Chapter 1 discusses the pre-consultation period with reference to the environment. The prepared nurse will offer a more efficient and effective consultation than one who has not considered environmental factors. There are many simple areas that can be addressed which can improve the ensuing consultation.

The most important part of a consultation is effective communication. This is the key to a satisfactory consultation for both the patient and the nurse. This includes the welcome, the nurse/patient relationship and observance of body language. Body language and active listening can be learned techniques. Chapter 2 uses scenarios to place communication skills into context within nursing practice. The advantages and disadvantages of telephone and email consultations are discussed within this chapter, but also referred to in later chapters. Aspects of all these skills are included throughout the text.

The principles of ethics are integral to all patient consultations. This includes confidentiality and consent, autonomy and advocacy. Chapter 3 aims to provide the reader with an insight into some of the issues that may be encountered during any consultation. Accurate and comprehensive documentation is explored. Aspects of the ethical issues discussed will be found throughout the book.

The Calgary-Cambridge consultation guide (Silverman et al, 2005) is adapted and expanded:in Chapter 4 but follows a basic framework. This relates to initiating the session, gathering information, physical examination, explanation and planning and closing the session. Chapter 4 examines the patient-centred consultation from welcome to closure. Although a medical model, it is easily adapted to nursing consultations. Nurses prepare for the consultation, establish a rapport with the patient, identify the reason for the consultation, consult, make an action plan and close the session. This occurs in all consultations, from administering a contraceptive injection to managing a leg ulcer.

Children and adolescent patients present unique challenges to the nursing consultation. It is important to gain an accurate understanding of the child's perspective of their condition. They are experts on themselves and only they can provide certain information. Chapter 5 examines some of the ethical and legal issues relating to this patient group, explores key issues with consultation skills and offers suggestions for management of some common scenarios.

The term disability covers a multitude of conditions, including physical, intellectual, visual and hearing impairment. Chapter 6 offers an insight into some of the challenges presented during a consultation, with tips for effecting a satisfactory and safe consultation. Issues of sexuality and cultural diversity within the disability framework are briefly discussed within the text.

Providing equitable health services demands that provision is appropriate, sensitive and inclusive. Research from Stonewall (2006) suggests that the gay population do not receive the same health care as the heterosexual population and are stigmatised due to their sexuality. Chapter 7 examines the experiences of lesbian, bisexual, gay and transgender (LBGT) patients to highlight good practice consultation skills in this marginalised population.

Understanding the challenges of delivering bad news to a patient is an important part of the nurse consultation as they will most likely encounter this situation on a regular basis. People differ in their perception of bad news. Bad news for one person can be good news for another. For example, a diagnosis of anaemia might be a relief for a patient who has been feeling tired and unwell for some weeks or months and was frightened in case the symptoms signified cancer. A diagnosis of diabetes can be devastating for a patient whose father had an amputation due to the disease. The do's and dont's of delivering bad news are discussed in Chapter 8. It is acknowledged that this skill, along with supporting patients and carers, usually develops with practice.

Nurses need to have an understanding of the cultural diversity of their practice population to be able to engage their patients during a consultation. This includes understanding the specific health problems of certain groups and their underlying health beliefs (Dhami and Sheikh, 2008). Chapter 9 offers guidance on consultation skills where ethnicity and culture may be a challenge within the practice. There is no emphasis on a particular culture but the examples are intended to highlight major issues. The reader is recommended to explore transcultural issues related to their practice population.

Chapters 1 to 9 explore and discuss various consultation skills. It is hoped that every reader will identify at least one area in the text where they can improve their skills. Chapter 10 offers a range of suggestions for developing these skills, from reflection to video recording a consultation.

The following comments were from seven people (two men, five women) aged 32-67 years whom I met in 2008, and illustrate positive and negative consultation experiences.

'I planned my travel in advance and the nurse was very helpful.'
'The nurse was very busy.'
'The nurse was on time.'
'I don't care what she looks like. I want the nurse to know what she is doing.'
'I appreciate time spent asking about my general health.'
'If there's a student present it's hard to say no. The student should be outside when the nurse asks.'
'I like an informal approach, with the patient in control, not being dictated to. A two-way consultation.'
'I want advice to be constant and correct. Three people in three surgeries all gave different advice.'
'Continuity of care is appreciated.'
'I get cross if kept waiting.'
'I had to pressurise the nurse to take my blood pressure.'
'The nurse took my blood pressure as routine.'
'If there's bad news I want it straight out in layman's terms, not on the telephone.'
'When I went for travel advice I had a full risk assessment.'

This book attempts to cover the management of most of the issues raised. Consultation skills for managing patients with mental health problems has been deliberately omitted as this requires more specialist skills.

There is inevitably an overlap of issues throughout the book. This should be viewed as reinforcement and not duplication. The reader will probably be able to relate to many of the scenarios cited within the text. Most are related to true incidents, although names have been changed for reasons of confidentiality, and some are hypothetical.

Consultation skills can be learned but we all need to identify our deficiencies. Researching and writing this book has been an enlightening process for the author.

Department of Health (2003) *Building on the best: choice, responsiveness and equity in the NHS. London.* The Stationery Office.

Dhami S & Sheikh A (2008) Health promotion: reaching ethnic minorities. *Practice Nurse.* **36**(8): 21-5

Kaufman G (2008) Patient assessment: effective consultation and history taking. *Nursing Standard.* **23**(4): 50-6

Kennedy I (2001) *Learning from Bristol: the Report of the Public Inquiry into children's heart surgery at the Bristol Royal Infirmary.* London: The Stationery Office: 280

Royal College of Nursing (2008) *'Dignity: at the heart of everything we do'* campaign. London. RCN

Silverman J, Kurtz S, Draper J (2005) *Skills for Communicating with Patients.*2nd Ed. Oxford. Radcliffe Publishing

Stonewall (2006) *Women and general health needs*

www.stonewall.org.uk/information_bank accessed 2/9/2006

CHAPTER I

The pre-consultation

This first chapter explores planning the consultation environment for maximum efficacy. When does the consultation start? Is it when the patient books into the surgery, or is it when he sits down in the consulting room? When does it end? Is it when the patient leaves the room, or is it when problems relating to the consultation, such as making a referral, have been dealt with?

Patients sometimes seek out nurses as their first point of contact because they are often perceived to have more time, expertise, and an in-depth knowledge of the patient's history (Brant, 2007). This is probably more common for minor injuries, chronic disease management and women's health. However, practice nurses see patients for many reasons.

Each consultation is individual and should be managed differently. For example, women coming for routine contraceptive reviews are usually relaxed and the consultation is simple, whereas a man attending for a blood test for suspected prostatic problems may be very anxious. Every consultation is different, yet they all start from the same basis.

First impressions

Dress
Miles (2008) stresses the importance of first impressions. Patients notice the nurses' appearance and the environment in which they work. A professional approach is essential to gain patient confidence. Although no one wishes to go back to regimented dress codes, professional dress, hair and jewellery code have their role in reducing cross infection.

Preparation
Be prepared for the consultation. Do not complete the previous patient's notes as the next one enters the room.

Try to establish the reason for a patient's appointment. For example, the appointment list may read: 'Margaret G, smear'. This offers the opportunity to note the previous smear history and gather cervical smear equipment together before the patient is called. However, the list is not always correct, and might read: 'Jim J, hep A', when he has in fact attended for a hepatitis B booster. This cannot always be avoided.

The patient could be surprised and pleased when you cite previous history, as they appreciate the nurse's knowledge and interest.

Refocus

Consultations can be challenging and emotionally draining. An example of a challenging consultation would be offering weight management support to someone whom has no motivation but knows they must lose weight before they can undergo important surgery. Also, a patient with a leg ulcer who interferes with the dressings can also frustrate the nurse. However, you must deal with any negative feelings or stress before the next patient consultation. Take a break or speak to a colleague to refocus for the next patient.

Starting the consultation

Calling the patient

Having checked the appointment list and the patient's records, it is now time to call them to the nurse's room. Each practice will have its own system of calling patients to a consulting room. These include calling via an intercom, a receptionist directing the patient, or the health professional going to the waiting room to collect their patient. There is no right or wrong way, but there are advantages and disadvantages to all methods.

The intercom

Advantages
- Saves nurse time collecting the patient
- Allows the nurse time to complete the notes from the previous patient and check the records of the next patient.

Disadvantages
- Is very impersonal
- The nurse cannot see the patient and assess their mobility
- A person with a hearing loss or who does not understand English may miss the call
- A wheelchair user might not be able to negotiate doors
- The patient may need assistance.

Receptionist directing the patient

Advantages
- Saves nurse time collecting the patient
- Allows nurse time to check the records while waiting for the patient
- A patient unfamiliar with the practice will be directed to the right room
- This is a more personal approach than being called by an intercom
- The receptionist could assist a patient if required
- Reduces the chance of a patient missing his appointment.

Disadvantages
- The nurse cannot see the patient and assess their mobility
- If the reception is busy there might not be staff available, which delays the patient consultation.

The nurse collecting her own patients

Advantages
- This is the most personal approach
- A patient is less likely to miss his appointment
- Gait and mobility can be assessed
- The patient walking with crutches or a wheelchair user can be assisted if required
- Leaving the room is good for time management, as it allows the nurse to regain her thoughts, and be ready for the next patient
- Walking to collect patients could be a source of exercise to practice nurse.

Disadvantages
- This approach can involve a lot of walking during the day!
- The time could be spent preparing for the consultation.

Scenario 1 puts this in perspective.

Establishing rapport and terms of address

Establishing rapport with the patient is a vital part of a successful consultation, and a crucial part of this rapport is empathy (Richards and Gregory 2005, Kaufman, 2008).

An important aspect of building rapport is knowing how to address the patient — should you call him Mr Jenkins or Joe? Older patients were brought up to call their friends and neighbours by their last names and might consider it disrespectful to be addressed by their first name. The patient may have a preference for the use of a first or last name, or may be ambivalent about how they are addressed. Only 77 of 475 patients in a study of patients consulting their GPs disliked being called by their first name, most of who were aged over 65 years (McKinstry, 1990). Many patients commented it helped put them at ease with the doctor. Although an old study relating to doctors, this is transferable to the practice nurse. Gillette et al (1992) concluded that it is difficult to predict reliably how a new patient will prefer to be addressed, but the majority of established patients will want to be called by their first names. More recent research supports these older studies (Makoul et al, 2007). Silverman et al (2005) advise that on meeting the patient you should consider how you carry out the following:

• Greeting the patient
• Introducing yourself
• Clarifying your role
• Obtaining the patient's name
• Demonstrating interest and respect
• Attending to the patient's physical comfort.

The manner of address will vary considerably depending on various factors. These include:

• Age of patient (as noted above)
• Knowing the person through school or socially
• The patient might have been seen every week for wound management over the past year
• How comfortable the nurse feels with the patient.

Some patients can appear over familiar and make the nurse uncomfortable. Using a first name might encourage this familiarity. Children are invariably addressed by their first name. Also, ensure the patient is aware of your name and role — it is very important to introduce yourself when you greet the patient.

The first greeting used in this scenario is more informal and will suit some patients, whereas the second is slightly more formal. Checking the spoken name with patient records can reduce mistaken identity and is fundamental to patient safety (Makoul et al, 2007). This is particularly important when father and son are both called John, or more than one patient has the same first and surnames, for example, Margaret Williams.

Anecdotally, regular patients prefer to be called by their first name, often stating that being called 'Mrs...' makes them feel old. Conversely, some patients call me Sister, Sister Mandy or Mandy. I encourage informality, but

Scenario 1

Mrs S is booked for a dressing. You have not seen her before. From the three methods of calling the patient described above, which one would you choose if you had the option?

Consider that you decided to collect her from the waiting room. When you call her name, an elderly lady struggles to stand up using two crutches. She is unaccompanied. What do you do next?

1. You direct her to your room while you leave a message at the reception desk. When you go back to your room, Mrs S is standing outside. The doors were too heavy for her to manage on her crutches.

2. You delay leaving a message at reception and assist Mrs S by opening all the doors and ensuring she can manage to be seated safely.

Having visually assessed Mrs S, it was obvious she was unable to manage to reach your room unaided. How would she have coped if called to the room via an intercom? This scenario can be transferred to all patients with a physical or learning disability. (See later chapter).

Scenario 2

A new patient attends for a health check following registration. You meet him in the waiting room and walk with him to your room. How do you start the consultation?

Nurse: 'Hello Mr Rogers. Please sit down. I'm Mandy and I'm a nurse practitioner, one of three nurses in the practice.'

Patient: 'Hello. If you're Mandy, then I'm Stan.'

Or

Nurse: 'Good morning, Mr Jones. Please sit down. I'm Sister Edwards.'

Patient: 'Good morning Sister.'

answer to anything. Do not assume that all patients who have been registered with the practice for years know your name. A patient recently asked me '*Are you new?*' My response was that I had been here for the last 19 years! Our paths just had not crossed over the years.

Developing a rapport with the patient includes being professionally friendly, showing an interest in the patient as a person and not as a condition, and actively using both verbal and non-verbal communication skills (see chapter 2). Patients should feel that staff are pleased to see them (Miles, 2008) — this includes the patients that you hoped would fail to attend! Greetings create a first impression, so forget the backlog of patients, smile and say '*Good morning, Mrs Brown*', and ensure patients know who you are. Not everyone will read your name badge.

The environment

The first part of most patient interactions is the preparation of the environment (Lloyd and Craig, 2007). The environment should be accessible, appropriately equipped, free from distractions and safe for the patient and nurse. Ideally the environment will be quiet with no interruptions. Privacy and dignity are also very important. The possibility of being overheard can discourage or prevent patients from disclosing information. Although the workplace should be inviting (Miles, 2008), in reality nurses have to work in whatever accommodation they are given. This may be a spacious office with all mod cons, or a small room with minimal facilities.

Patient comfort is also important, as illustrated in *Box 1.1*. Issues to consider whatever the accommodation are noted in *Figure 1.1* and *Box 1.1*.

- Think about the environment in which you work. Is there sufficient seating? Although the couch can be regarded as a seat, it is preferable to collect another chair for a companion, especially if they require assistance. Are the chairs comfortable? Can they be washed?
- A messy room suggests a messy nurse. An uncluttered room can look either professional or cold. A photo on the desk is often an easy way to make the room more personal and can help create a rapport with the patient
- Ensure there is room for both the wheelchair user and the carer, if appropriate. This might necessitate removing a chair from the room
- Reassure the patient that all steps are taken to ensure privacy
- Do not expect the patient to have to leave their clothes on the floor. Ideally a hanger or hooks would be available. Alternatively ensure a chair is available
- It can be difficult to prevent being overheard, especially if the patient talks loudly. Ensure the door is firmly closed so that noise is muffled to preserve confidentiality

---

Box 1.1 The environment

1. How are the desk and chairs positioned? Is there a barrier between the nurse and the patient?
2. Is the room cluttered?
3. Is there room for a relative or carer to be present in the room and are they seated in an appropriate position, especially if they are involved in the consultation? Is there room to manoeuvre a wheelchair?
4. Do the blinds close? Are there curtains around the couch? Does the door lock?
5. Is there somewhere for the patient to place their clothes?
6. Can the consultation be overheard?
7. Is the room cold, or hot and stuffy?
8. Is outside noise, such as traffic, a distraction?
9. Is there an escape route?

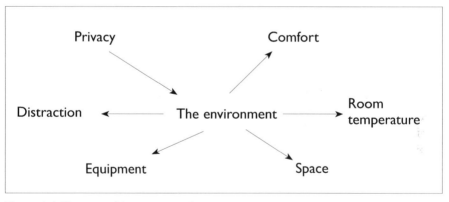

Figure 1.1 The consulting room environment.

- Everyone interprets temperature differently. Try to adapt to individual needs, including your own
- Closing windows and doors can reduce noise, while room temperature should be comfortable for both the nurse and patient
- For safety reasons, the nurse should be nearest to the door to enable a quick exit in case of violence or abuse. In practical terms this is not always possible, so the nurse must be aware of risk, inviting a colleague to be in the room during the consultation if necessary. Ideally each consulting room will have an alarm system for the nurse to call for assistance in case of emergency.

Some of these issues are discussed more fully in other chapters.

Equip for purpose

The room should be equipped for purpose. Check the appointment list whenever possible and prepare the equipment accordingly. Ensure all expected injections are in the room but stored out of patient sight. These might include B12, contraceptive or hormonal injections. These should be returned to a lockable cupboard if the patient fails to attend. However, vaccines should be maintained within the cold chain, and only taken from the fridge when required (DH, 2006).

There should be sufficient cervical smear equipment to hand so the nurse does not have to leave the woman on the couch while she goes in search of a larger or smaller speculum.

A patient attending for a regular dressing might bring his dressings at every visit, or they may be stored in a central area in the surgery. Collect these before the patient arrives to save time. A wound should not be left uncovered whilst searching for a dressing.

Interruptions

Ideally there should be no interruptions during a consultation (Edwards, 2008). Intra-practice telephone calls should be used only when essential. Reception staff need to be trained not to transfer patient queries for travel advice or baby immunisations to the nurse during a consultation — these can be managed by the patient details being noted and dealt with when the nurse is free. Any interruption can result in the patient or nurse losing their concentration (see Chapter 4).

Privacy

The consulting environment should encourage trust, confidence and facilitate talking (Robertson, 2008).The need to consider patient privacy cannot be overstated. For example, explain to a woman that you are locking the consulting room door before undertaking a cervical smear for her privacy as patients tend to confuse room numbers, and colleagues might be looking for equipment such as dressings.

It can be argued that patients who attend mass influenza clinics are denied privacy. Efforts must be made to ensure privacy even for this apparently innocuous intervention.

Scenario 3

A 29-year-old woman attends for a smear, having been allocated a 10 minute appointment. The nurse greets her by name, introduces herself and asks her to be seated. The consultation goes as follows:

Nurse: 'What can I do for you today?' (Does not assume that the appointment documentation is correct.)

Miss P: 'I've come for my smear.'

Nurse: 'Can you tell me what you understand by a smear?'

Miss P: 'It's to check for cancer.'

Nurse: 'Lots of women think that, but it's actually to check for abnormal cells. If these are monitored and treated, it would be unusual to develop cancer.'

Miss P: 'Some of my friends have had treatment.'

The nurse then asks about contraception, periods, and assesses the risk of sexually transmitted infections as she completes the smear form.

Nurse: 'What's your partner's name?' (Does not assume heterosexuality.)

Miss P: 'It was Tom, but we split up two months ago after I found he's been unfaithful.'

Nurse: 'Would you like to talk about it?'

Miss P briefly describes the breakdown.

Nurse: 'Would you like me to take some swabs to check for infection?'

Miss P: 'Oh yes please. I've been really worried.'

The nurse then allows Miss P to undress in privacy while she prepares the swab forms, gains informed consent, takes vaginal and endocervical swabs and smear, and discusses the results before Miss P leaves the room. The nurse advises Miss P to attend the genito-urinary clinic for a full screen, giving written contact details.

The length of appointments

Time constraints usually limit the length of a consultation, but there are techniques for maximising the quality of the consultation. Insufficient time can result in incomplete information that may adversely affect the patient's care (Lloyd and Craig, 2007). It is important not to appear rushed, even when you are, as this may interfere with the patient's willingness to disclose vital information. Women's health can also be fraught with problems. Open questions allow the patient to set the agenda and improve the quality of the consultation, but can overrun the allocated time.

This consultation in scenario 3 took 20 minutes. It could be undertaken in 10 minutes if no questions are asked, but would that have been a satisfactory consultation for the patient? It is important that a patient understands what an abnormal smear result actually means, and also Miss P might not have volunteered the information that suggested she might be at risk of a sexually transmitted infection unless prompted.

The reader can probably relate this scenario to numerous occasions in her own practice. Nurses are accountable for their acts and omissions. If a consultation is rushed and vital information is not disclosed or recorded, they can then be liable for a claim of negligence (NMC, 2008).

If there is insufficient time for a particular type of consultation, raise this issue with management. For example, a 10 minute appointment for a new patient registration will be ample for a young, fit 20-year-old, but does not allow sufficient time to address the initial requirements of the diabetic patient with co-morbidity and three sheets of repeat prescriptions. Negotiate with the practice manager and ensure reception staff are aware of how much time is required for a particular routine task. There will, of course, be occasions when this does not run to plan. There is no need to extend a consultation beyond the planned task, unless clinically indicated, although social interaction can improve patient and nurse satisfaction. If a task is completed in five minutes, this allows five minutes to catch breath and prepare for the next patient.

What do you do when a patient arrives late for their appointment? Consider the four options below. Do you:

- Squeeze them in between booked patients
- Ask them to wait until you are free
- Ask them to re-book
- Send them to a colleague?

This can be a difficult issue to address. There may be a legitimate reason for the delay, for example traffic problems or a family crisis. However, it could also be that the patient turns up when they feel like it.

Good consultation skills are essential in these cases, and also you must give consideration to what treatment the patient is booked for. If it is, for example, a suture removal, which is usually simple and quick, there might be other concerns the patient wishes to raise such as postoperative recovery. In this case, it may be necessary to initially state that you only have 5 minutes and can undertake suture removal but ask the patient to re-book if he/she wants to discuss other issues. Alternatively, a consultation on diet advice is not urgent and can be sensitively rebooked. The nurse must use her skills to assess each situation. For example, I always find time for my 80-year-old patient who is a week late for his B12 injection.

What about the patient's time?

It must not be forgotten that patients also have to manage their time. Their commitments may include work, other medical appointments, family, or social issues. Although they like to be seen quickly for their appointments, patients like the nurse to have plenty of time to listen to their problems. If the nurse runs behind with her appointments, people usually respond well to a simple '*I'm sorry to have kept you waiting*' and a thorough consultation. The nurse who regularly falls behind with booked appointments may need to reassess her time management. Time spent in the initial patient consultation may reduce subsequent consultations.

If several issues can be dealt with during one consultation, future appointments can be saved, which benefits both nurse and patient in regard to time management (Edwards, 2008). Longer appointments are often required for patients with special needs, including ethnic minorities, those with a hearing loss who require an interpreter, and those with physical and learning disabilities. This is discussed in Chapters 7 and 9.

Scenario 4 overleaf places time management and accountability in context. This scenario highlights the importance of considering all aspects of a patient's health, and not merely treating the patient as a condition. Although time was limited, the extra few minutes spent recording the blood pressure and arranging routine blood tests was time well spent. The respiratory aspect proved to be second in importance to the renal function. The Code (NMC, 2008) also states that the nurse is answerable for her actions and omissions. It could be argued that not taking a blood pressure could be viewed as an omission.

It can be difficult to know whether or not you do the patient a favour by identifying a potentially serious condition. However, Mrs A telephoned the surgery following her urology appointment to thank the nurse for identifying the problem. The cancer was surgically removed and Mrs A's breathlessness resolved spontaneously.

Scenario 4

Mrs A is a 68-year-old woman with a history of nephrectomy for carcinoma of the kidney and chronic fatigue syndrome. She was referred to the practice nurse for respiratory assessment and spirometry following a chest X-ray suggestive of chronic obstructive pulmonary disease. Assessment identified an MRC dyspnoea scale of 3–4 (where 1 is good and 5 is housebound), with shortness of breath that Mrs A associated with her chronic fatigue. The nurse took the opportunity to follow up a previous raised blood pressure and gained Mrs A's permission to arrange routine blood tests including full blood count and thyroid function to exclude anaemia or thyroid disease as causes of breathlessness, and renal function. The blood results highlighted a urea of 21.5 (normal range 1.0-7.0 mmol/L), creatinine 321 (normal range 60-120 mmol/L), and eGFR of 13 (normal >90mL/min), suggestive of chronic kidney disease (CKD) stage 5.

Although Mrs A attended for a respiratory assessment, the experienced nurse undertook a holistic approach that included all aspects of her current health. The nurse took the opportunity to re-check her blood pressure, which highlighted borderline hypertension that required investigation. The investigations were consistent with CKD 5. Other blood tests were reported as normal.

Following a repeat blood test that confirmed abnormal kidney function, Mrs A was referred urgently for urological assessment. An MRI scan showed an occlusive transitional cell carcinoma (TCC) obstructing the remaining ureter. Surgery was planned to excise the ureteric carcinoma.

The practice nurse might have concentrated solely on the referral for respiratory assessment during the 20-minute appointment, in which case the blood pressure would not have been rechecked, investigations instigated or the abnormal results identified. Subsequently the ureteric obstruction would not have been diagnosed, which in turn could have resulted in deterioration in Mrs A's health until the carcinoma was inoperable.

Timed appointments are for the benefit of the patient and the nurse. However, there are occasions when it is in the patient's interest to extend a consultation. Time management is very important, but many patients benefit from a more thorough consultation. If the nurse is running behind with her appointments, it is good manners to let patients know there is a delay, so they can re-book if they prefer. However, for those patients who never seem to want to go home, a pre-arranged telephone call from a colleague, or a knock on the door, can hasten the conclusion of an overlong consultation.

Summary

Some patients are more concerned with their nursing care and management than the environment. However, take time to review the working environment for health and safety risks, comfort and privacy. Stock the room before surgery commences. Think about how to welcome your patients. Introduce yourself to new patients and let them know how you like to be addressed. This is as important as the manner in which they are addressed when developing the nurse-patient rapport. Consider the timing of appointments, flexibility, but most importantly, your accountability. Is there time to undertake the task safely and effectively? If not, negotiate this with management.

Key points

- Welcome the patient with a smile
- Prepare the room
- Consider time management from both the nurse and patient perspectives

Brant C (2007) The nurse will see you. *Nursing Standard* **22**(13): 62–3

Department of Health (2006) *Immunisation Against Infectious Diseases* 3rd edn. The Stationery Office, London

Edwards M (2008) *The Informed Practice Nurse* 2nd edn. Wiley, Chichester

Gillette RD, Filak A, Thorne C (1992) First name or last name: which do patients prefer? *Journal Board Family Practice* **5**(5): 517–22

Kaufman G (2008) Patient assessment: effective consultation and history taking. *Nursing Standard* **23**(4): 50–6

Lloyd H, Craig S (2007) A guide to taking a patient's history. *Nursing Standard* **22**(13): 42–8

Makoul G, Zick A, Green M (2007) An Evidence-based Perspective on Greetings in Medical Encounters. *Archives of Internal Medicine* **167**(11): 1171–6

Miles J (2008) Effective communication. *Practice Nurse* **35**(2): 42–7

McKinstry B (1990) Should general practitioners call patients by their first names? *British Medical Journal* **301**: 795–6

Nursing and Midwifery Council (2008) *The Code. Standards of conduct, performance and ethics for nurses and midwives.* NMC, London

Richards S, Gregory S (2005) Developing consultation skills. *Practice Nurse* **29**(11): 13–20

Robertson K (2008) The importance of communication skills. *BMJ Learning. Practice Nurse CPD*. http://learning.bmj.com accessed 20/10/2008

Silverman J, Kurtz S, Draper J (2005) *Skills for Communicating with Patients* 2nd edn. Radcliffe Publishing, Oxford

CHAPTER 2

Communication skills

Everyone communicates in some manner, whether verbally, physically or on paper. Communication skills are a vital tool for all health workers to avoid conveying inadvertent messages about our attitudes, our feelings, our beliefs, our assumptions and our prejudices (Robertson, 2008). It is not possible to satisfy all patients all of the time, however satisfaction has been linked to empathy, non-judgmental attitude and warm non-verbal communication (Robertson, 2008). Poor communication can affect the patient's attitude and understanding of their condition. This can lead to confusion or poor concordance with treatment, resulting in wasted medication and poorer health outcomes. It can also lead to dissatisfaction on behalf of both patients and nurses. There are also occasions when a patient has not fully understood the doctor, and makes an appointment with the nurse for a clearer explanation.

This chapter will examine different ways of communication to help nurses make the most of their consultation skills. Overlap of certain points will reinforce important issues. For simplicity, the term concordance has been used to include compliance and adherence.

Clinical competence

There are different forms of communication. One that may be overlooked is physical appearance. Nurses who project professionalism during the consultation are more likely to gain patients' confidence in their clinical competencies. Untidiness or slovenliness will communicate a negative image to the patient. Patients are also reassured when the nurse refers to a textbook or internet to reinforce her knowledge, especially if they can say 'That spot looks like impetigo', and then shows the patient a photograph in a dermatology book.

Positioning

In all consultations it is important to consider the patient/nurse space. The patient will not be comfortable if the nurse is standing whilst they are sitting. Level eye contact is ideal where possible. It can also be impersonal talking to the patient from the other side of the room. Sitting face-on to the patient can appear threatening, while sitting square-on is more personal. A desk between nurse and patient is a major barrier to the nurse/patient relationship, as is the patient being too close to the nurse. This is discussed later in this chapter.

Confidentiality

One area of confidentiality that is sometimes difficult to control is unavoidably sharing information. This can occur through closed doors when a patient is hard of hearing. He/she may shout, and the nurse has to raise her voice to be heard. In an ideal situation the nurse will speak quietly but audibly. Playing music in the waiting room or corridor can help mask consultations.

Responding skills

Robertson (2008) describes responding skills involved in patient consultations. The four skills relevant to nurses are:
- Attending
- Following
- Questioning
- Reflecting.

Attending skills

These are non-verbal behaviours that indicate interest and attention, and include:

- An open posture, facing, leaning slightly on to the patient
- Appropriate body movement and distance from the patient
- Appropriate eye contact, being aware of cultural norms (see Chapter 9)
- An open facial expression, appropriately responsive to the patient's story.

Paying close attention to the patient's non-verbal behaviour will improve the nurse's own ability to communicate non-verbally. It is also important to identify if the patient's words do not match the non-verbal behaviour. For example, a patient might state he is 'fine' but avoids eye contact, or his eyes start to water. Eye contact lasting four to five seconds is recommended, while it can appear threatening if it lasts longer.

Following skills

Non-verbal cues can be misunderstood. For example, anger might not be directed at the nurse. A patient might appear cross that they have been kept waiting when the real cause is that the central heating engineer failed to fix the boiler. The following scenarios are examples of different following skills.

Patients vary in their needs. One patient might not wish to share their grief and prefer to 'get on with it', while another will need a shoulder to cry on. The nurse needs to take the cue from the patient.

Verbal and non-verbal encouragers indicate that the nurse is listening, interested and following what the patient is saying (see *Box 2.1*). Probes are open-ended requests for elaborating on an issue. They also reassure the patient that the nurse is listening to their concerns. Attentive listening is both active and highly skilled (Silverman et al, 2005). The skills needed to listen attentively include wait time, facilitative response, non-verbal skills and picking up verbal and non-verbal cues. Attentive silence, or wait time, can be one of the most powerful communication skills (Robertson, 2008). It allows

---

Scenario 1

Mrs W attends for her routine smear. She is visibly upset when she enters the room. The nurse has 10 minutes for the smear so begins to ask the relevant questions to complete the documentation. She asks Mrs W what has upset her, and learns that her best friend has been diagnosed with breast cancer. The nurse says how sorry she is to hear this, hands her a tissue, and then directs her to the couch for the procedure. When finished she explains how the smear results will be received, says goodbye, and sees the patient out of the room.

Scenario 2

Mrs W attends for her routine smear. She is visibly upset when she enters the room. The nurse has 10 minutes for the smear. Before she starts completing the smear documentation she asks Mrs W what has upset her and learns that her best friend has been diagnosed with breast cancer. The nurse puts down her pen, puts the tissue box on the desk and listens while Mrs W talks about her feelings. This is her third friend with cancer, one of whom died earlier that year. Mrs W shares her feelings and concerns with the nurse, who suggests the smear is taken another time when there is more time and Mrs W feels better.

---

the patient to think and try to decide how to respond. When the patient is distressed, silence can allow them to think about their distress and regain their composure rather than distract them (see Scenario 2). It can convey support and comfort. *Boxes 2.2* and *2.3* list some of the elements of attentive and non-listening communication.

Box 2.1 Verbal and non-verbal encouragers

Non verbal   **Verbal**
Eye contact   Verbal prompts, such as: 'Aha…hmmm…'
Interested posture
Head nods
Hand gestures
Facial gestures

Box 2.2 Attentive listening

Sounds like   **Looks like**
'Tell me that again'   Nodding
'I know what you mean'   Making eye contact
'Tell me more'   Positive body language
'What you're saying is…'   Smiling

Box 2.3 Non-listening

Sounds like   **Looks like**
Tapping pencil   Darting eyes
Winding watch   Fidgeting
Saying: 'Uh huh' a lot   Playing with hair
Saying: 'Really'   Turning away
Sighing   Looking at clock

Questioning skills

Questions can be open-ended, closed or focused. Consultations often require a mix of questions. Find out what the patient believes to be their problems and how these affect their life.

Open questions
Open questions allow greater exploration of an issue, for example: '*Tell me more about the headache*', or '*Describe the discharge*'. The patient perspective can be ascertained by asking them about their concerns. Prompts are helpful for encouraging the patient to expand these concerns. Open-ended questions take up more time in the consultation as the patient elaborates on his condition or concern, especially if talkative, but allow a deeper understanding of the patient's concerns.

Closed questions
Closed questions will usually result in a simple 'Yes/No' answer and offers little information, unless the patient is particularly vocal. For example: '*Do you take your inhaler every day?*' is a closed question, while: '*When did you last use your inhaler?*' allows the patient to elaborate. Closed questions can be useful to elicit particular details, for example: '*Do you bleed between your periods?*'. If the answer is 'yes', this can be explored further. Allow the patient time to answer. Closed questions can be useful when time is limited.

Focused questions
Focused questions allow the nurse to gain specific information by narrowing the line of questioning. Scenario 3 overleaf places these questions in context during one consultation:

Unhelpful question types
Leading questions and compound questions are unhelpful question types that are better avoided. Leading questions suggest the desired answer and are difficult for the patient to disagree with. For example: '*You don't cough at night, do you?*' is likely to elicit a 'no' response, whereas: '*When did you last have a night cough?*' allows the patient to elaborate.

Compound questions confuse both patient and nurse, as the patient cannot answer all questions at the same time, and the nurse is unsure which question has been answered. For example: '*Do you have any pain, discharge or bleeding after intercourse?*'. If the woman says 'yes' the nurse will have to break down the list to clarify the symptom.

Scenario 3

Nurse: 'What can I do for you today?' (open question)

Patient: 'I've tried to diet but need some help.'

Nurse: 'Tell me what you've tried in the past.' (focused question to help elaborate)

Patient: 'I've tried all the slimming clubs, I lose weight but then put it back on.'

Nurse: 'Would you like me to weigh you today, and we can plan what support I can offer you?' (closed question to gain a 'yes/no' answer)

Patient: 'Yes please.'

Backtracking extends the consultation, therefore ask each question individually and allow the patient time to answer.

The tone of voice can convey a wealth of information, ranging from enthusiasm to disinterest. Use the tone of voice to emphasise particular ideas. Express enthusiasm using an animated tone of voice. The nurse who appears disinterested is unlikely to gain the necessary rapport for an effective consultation.

Reflecting skills

Reflecting skills enable the nurse to let the patient know they are listening and have understood their perspective. Paraphrasing is the repetition of words in a slightly different format to check the information has been correctly interpreted. Go over what the patient has said from time to time to check you understand what the patient means.

Empathy is another powerful communication skill — when the patient feels the nurse acknowledges the emotional content. Summarising from the patient's point of view can be a way of expressing empathy. Scenario 4 shows reflecting skills in practice.

In general, all these techniques improve the performance of someone who is interested and cares about them. They cannot be `switched on' at will, as the patient can tell the difference and not respond positively to indifference.

Scenario 4

Patient: 'I know I should stop smoking, what with my asthma and the kids getting at me, and I can't afford it. I've tried to give up before, but started again when the wife was ill. I really need to stop.'

Nurse: 'It sounds like you would like to give up smoking with some help.' (paraphrasing)

Patient: 'I do want to stop, but it's hard…what with the worry about job losses.'

Nurse: 'I can understand that you are worried about your job. I read about it in the paper.' (empathy)

Patient: 'My breathing's been bad for the last two weeks, my inhaler doesn't help much. I've got to do something.'

Nurse: 'It is hard to stop smoking, but it would help your breathing and we can offer you help with this.' (summarising)

Giving information

Information should be delivered in chunks, reiterated and reinforced at subsequent consultations as there is often too much to assimilate at one time. This also reassures the nurse that the patient has understood previous instructions or advice. Most patients do not understand technical language or jargon, and require the consultation to be clear and simple.

The other extreme is the patients who attend with their internet print out or graphs of their blood sugars or fat content of each meal. They might feel patronised if the nurse refers to the 'blue and brown' inhalers, rather than 'bronchodilator' and 'inhaled steroid inhalers'. This is the advantage of the nurse having a good relationship with her patients and speaking their language.

Better-informed patients have greater self-management. Those patients who attend with information about their condition and/or medications can improve the patient-centred consultation through their involvement in decision-making (see Chapter 4).

Scenario 5

Mr P had an appointment for ear irrigation before having a hearing aid fitted. The nurse welcomed him and offered him a seat. Having read the patient notes before calling Mr P, the nurse noted that the doctor prescribed Mr P medication for hypertension three months ago, but this has not been reviewed. After the initial chat, the nurse took Mr P's blood pressure. It was an average of 160/102 after three readings.

She had three options:

1. Ask the patient to have his blood pressure checked in a month
2. Ask the doctor to increase the medication
3. Take time to assess patient understanding and concordance

Option 1 would have left Mr P with no medication and the risk of cardiovascular disease resulting from uncontrolled hypertension.

Option 2 would have resulted in Mr P being over-treated, with the risk of hypotension or unpleasant side-effects of the medication.

The nurse chose Option 3. In this instance, Mr P was under the impression that the treatment was complete. He did not understand that treatment would probably be for life. He ran out of tablets two months ago and did not realise he needed a blood pressure check to assess his control. The nurse explained why the treatment was necessary, how it worked, potential side effects reinforced with a leaflet, and made Mr P a review appointment for one month. A further prescription for medication was generated.

Fortunately, Mr P did not require ear irrigation, as the drums were visible.

Advice for patients about medicines

One of the most significant effects of poor communication is confusion about medicines — when patients feel they do not know enough about the potential side effects and subsequent wastage of medicines (Prentice, 2008). Ensure the patient understands what the medicine is for, how it works, potential side effects and what to do if they have any concerns before they leave the room. This is a role for all nurses whether or not they are nurse prescribers. Scenario 5 places the importance of clear information in context.

It highlights the importance of ensuring patients are clear about how long long the medication is to be taken and when to return. Anecdotally, patients believe they will be cured with one prescription.

Patients should have the facility to telephone the practice with medication queries and either speak to, or leave a message for, the nurse who generated the prescription. However this is not always practical and it is reasonable to tell patients they can ask their pharmacist or contact NHS Direct if they have a question and the practice is busy (Prentice, 2008). This will relieve pressure on the practice and enable the patient to get all the advice they need as quickly as possible.

Signposting

Good consultation skills include knowing when the patient needs to be referred to a colleague within the practice or signposted to another agency. This could be a self-help group, or a charity offering advice. The Internet is a useful reference tool. Nurses can improve patients' knowledge about their disease by actively directing them to credible websites.

Alternatively, although there may be no time during the consultation, the nurse can offer to search for the information for the patient to collect later.

Listening skills

Active listening

At the start of the consultation allow the patient to talk without interruption. Most patients will have told the nurse everything relevant to their problem within two minutes. Once interrupted, patients rarely reintroduce a new issue, which can result in failure to disclose significant concerns.

Listening is one of the most important skills required during a consultation. This is a two way process, allowing the nurse to obtain information, and the patient to understand and learn. However, it is reported that only 25–50% of what is heard is remembered (Mind Tools, 2008). This has implications for both parties during a consultation. Has the nurse heard what the patient has said? Does the patient understand the lifestyle advice or self-management plan discussed by the nurse? See *Box 2.4* for non-verbal elements of active listening. Good listening skills can prevent conflict and misunderstandings. See *Box 2.5* and *2.6*.

Structured education, which gives patients information in small chunks to keep them interested, is discussed in Chapter 4.

Box 2.4 Non-verbal elements in active listening (SOLER)

- Sitting SQUARE on to the patient
- With an OPEN position
- LEANING slightly forward
- With EYE contact
- In a RELAXED posture

(Source: Kaufman 2008)

Box 2.5 Active listening skills

- Pay attention
- Use your body language to show you are listening
- Provide feedback during the consultation
- Allow the speaker to finish
- Summarise what the patient has said

Box 2.6 Examples of active listening skills

- Using open questions: 'You don't seem surprised by the result. Why is that?'
- Seeking elaboration: 'I see you are more breathless today. What does it prevent you doing?'
- Seeking specific examples: 'You're obviously bothered by this infection. How many times have you needed treatment?'

Box 2.7 Unhelpful consultation techniques

- Using technical or inappropriate jargon can confuse the patient
- Giving false reassurance can result in the patient losing confidence in the health professionals
- Jumping to conclusions can distract the patient
- Leading questions such as 'Do you cough in the morning?' can stifle patient expression

Scenario 6

Mr B attended for a pneumococcal injection. His computer records had an entry that this had been given in 2006. He was adamant that he had not received the vaccination. What would you do?

Options:

1. Refuse to give the injection as it was already recorded in his notes.
2. Think: 'Oh well', and give it anyway as it wouldn't hurt.
3. Listen to the patient, apologise for the misunderstanding, note the error in the patient records and give the injection.
4. Reassure the patient that the injection had been given.

Option 3 shows you are listening to your patient. He is likely to feel patronised if told he has had the injection, when he knows he has not. There are occasions, however, when a patient has a degree of dementia and forgets what they have had. In these instances it is safer to trust the patient's records!

Success in eliciting a patient's problems lies in active listening (Richards and Gregory, 2005). Spend an appropriate time listening and less time talking (Miles, 2008). The patient who attends for a postoperative dressing may have planned to discuss something totally unconnected with the booked appointment. Another patient may attend with a newspaper or internet report/scare that they wish to discuss and test the nurse's knowledge against the media. It is essential to consider what the patient wants from the consultation.

Examples of unhelpful interview techniques which are best avoided are listed in *Box 2.7*.

Pay attention to what the patient is saying and doing

In order to be an active listener it is necessary to pay careful attention to the patient. Try to maintain eye contact — it is impossible to give undivided attention to a patient whilst looking at a computer screen. If necessary, jot notes on a piece of paper and then expand when completing the documentation at the end of the consultation.

Loss of concentration will lead to loss of focus and contribute to a lack of listening and understanding. When the mind wanders try repeating the patient's words mentally as they speak to reinforce their message and reduce mind drift.

It can be difficult to pay attention when children are disruptive. Parents and grandparents often have young children with them, so diversionary tactics are useful. These can be by supplying (quiet) toys or drawing materials to entertain the child, allowing you to attend to the patient.

Environmental factors can also be distracting. These have been discussed in Chapter 1. Distraction with children present is discussed in Chapter 5.

Body language

Body language means communication with the movement or position of the human body, and can be conscious or unconscious. Body language is often a subconscious activity intended to create a balance between inner feelings and outer appearance. All aspects of body language relate to both the patient and the nurse (see *Figure 2.1*). Examples of body language are listed in *Box 2.8*. *Table 2.1* includes examples of positive and negative body language.

Nurses who have an increased awareness of their own body language have an increased ability to read other people's body language. Patients who are emotional might notice the smallest lapse of attention, or jump to the conclusion that the nurse is bored or feels they are a nuisance, which will compound their feeling of depression or low self-esteem. The speaker's face is the most reliable source of information about a person's mood. Awareness of body language enables the nurse to tell if a patient is happy, sad, sullen, irritated, bored or impatient.

Body language can be defensive or open; for example arms crossed across the chest are a defensive posture, whilst visible palms indicate openness and sincerity.

Appearance is also a means of communication. For example, what message does the unkempt patient send to the nurse? For this you have several options:
- Depressed and cannot be bothered
- Dementia and 'away with the fairies'
- Unaware due to cultural norms.

The nurse has to try to ascertain which category the patient fits into when trying to develop a rapport with the patient. Unfortunately, the offensive smelling patient may receive shorter consultations than necessary, and will receive inequitable care. This is a sensitive issue and difficult to resolve.

In another example, the patient who is looking at the wall is not interested in what the nurse is saying. In this case bring the patient back to the consultation by asking them to repeat in their own words what was just said, or terminate the consultation and document that the patient is unreceptive to health advice (see Chapter 3).

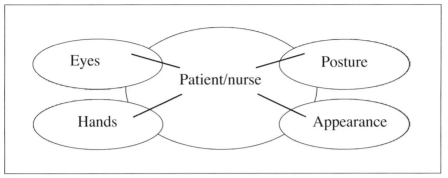

Figure 2.1 Key aspects of body language

Box 2.8 Body language

- The movement of arms and legs
- Body posture
- The manner of sitting
- Facial expressions
- Gait
- Eye movements
- Regular gestures such as stroking hair or touching the nose

---

Table 2.1 Examples of positive and negative body language.

Positive signs	Negative signs
Eye contact, but must not be overdone	Fiddling with hair suggests insecurity
Lounging with arms and legs dangling suggests the person is relaxed and feeling comfortable	Quickened breathing or clenched fists suggests tension
Smile with open lips and tilt the head slightly to show attentiveness (but not flirting)	Sitting on the edge of the chair with legs outstretched and feet crossed can signal indifference
Firm, friendly handshake when greeting the patient	Hands clasped behind the head suggests arrogance
Sitting with palms showing is an open posture	The patient who taps his feet, looks down, slouches or has his head in his hands is probably bored

Be aware of both your and the patient's body language. Use body language to shown the patient you are listening to them. This can be a nod of the head or an '*Uh huh*', which can encourage the patient to continue speaking and offer all the relevant information. Smile and use other facial expressions. A smile that does not reach the eyes sends signals of falseness and insecurity. Practice an open and inviting posture.

Provide feedback

It is essential to understand what has been said by the patient during the consultation. Reflect on what the patient has said to clarify a point and avoid a misunderstanding. Examples of questions used in reflection include, for example:

- '*What do you mean when you say you are short of breath?*'
- '*It sounds like you are saying you are worried about this discharge?*'
- '*Is this what you mean?*'

Feedback shows the patient that the nurse has been listening but that she needs a little more clarification. Do not make assumptions from a consultation that has not been comprehensive.

Allow the speaker to finish

Interrupting a consultation wastes time and frustrates the speaker. It can also lead to the patient losing their train of thought, which in turn may lead to the loss of relevant information. It has been suggested that many health professionals barely manage 20 seconds of listening before interrupting their patients (Miles, 2008). Allow the patient to finish speaking. However, there are patients who would never stop speaking, and in these instances it is necessary to focus the consultation to a key health concern.

Closing a consultation

The consultation needs a conclusion. What happens next? Does the patient need to be reviewed? If so, when and by whom? What medication does he/she need, how often does he take it, and does he take it for life? The following two scenarios are examples of appropriate closures.

Scenario 7

Mr S attended for a sick note following stripping of his varicose veins. The left groin wound has an offensive discharge, for which the doctor prescribed a five-day course of antibiotics. The doctor refers Mr S to the nurse for a dressing on Monday afternoon The nurse takes a swab, then cleans and dresses the wound. She explains how and why she is taking the swab, and when to expect the result. She also explains that the wound will need to be reviewed on Friday, and makes a convenient appointment. She ensures that Mr S understands the medication regime, reinforcing the need to complete the course of tablets. He was advised to contact the surgery if he had any concerns.

Closure: Mr S knew what medication he was taking, how often he would take it and for how many days. He knew when to return for a dressing change and why, but was reassured that he could contact the surgery at any time if he was worried about the wound.

Scenario 8

Jane is an 18-year-old girl who attends for contraceptive advice. She wants to start the same combined oral contraceptive pill as her friend. The nurse takes a full risk assessment to ascertain suitability for the combined pill and discusses all possible methods of contraception. During the assessment it transpires that Jane usually has a 28-day menstrual cycle, but is a day overdue this month. She has a regular partner and currently uses condoms for contraception, but thinks one might have split 10 days ago. Jane is a non-smoker with no contraindications to the pill. A pregnancy test taken in the surgery is negative. It is not appropriate to commence hormonal contraception until Jane has a menstrual period.

Closure: the nurse concludes the consultation by supplying Jane with a leaflet about all forms of contraception, including the combined pill, to ensure she is informed about long acting forms of contraception. She advises Jane to continue using condoms and return in a week for a further pregnancy test if she does not have her period. Jane is also advised to book an appointment with the doctor or nurse as soon as her period starts, so that the chosen method of contraception can be prescribed.

In this instance, Jane knew exactly what would happen next. She was to return for a pregnancy test and decide an action plan if she did not start her period within a given timescale. If she started her period then she would contact the surgery for an appointment to start her chosen method of contraception.

The management phase of consultations

The patient who has a clear understanding of their condition and how to manage it, both through lifestyle and through pharmacological means, is more likely to follow a recommended management plan (Robertson, 2008). Time, patience, supportive literature and empathy with the patient are all required to deliver information about the physiology of chronic disease such as asthma or diabetes, or for wound healing. In order to aid concordance, explain clearly and simply how treatment works and how to self-manage the condition (see *Table 2.2*).

Some patients wish to take their treatment with little explanation of cause and effect, and this non-autonomous attitude should be respected (Edwards, 2008). Also, consider those patients who cannot read, those with learning or visual disability and those for whom English is not the first language (see Chapters 6 and 9).

Table 2.2 Examples of explanations that can aid concordance.	
Condition	Explanation
Diabetes	Link between medication reducing high blood sugars and reducing subsequent organ damage
Asthma	Link between certain trigger factors and inflammation of the bronchioles, and the role of inhaled steroids to prevent inflammation
Warfarin	Adverse effect of alcohol with anticoagulants
Cellulitis	Necessity of high dose oral antibiotics to prevent septicaemia
Hypertension	Benefits of non-pharmacological management to reduce blood pressure without medication

Patient education and information giving

Although education and self-management have traditionally been considered necessary for some long term conditions, for example diabetes, it has been reported that these interventions have had discouraging results in reducing complications (Hornsten et al, 2005). The focus of education has changed from providing medical information by didactic teaching to assisting and strengthening patients to improve their self-management skills, self-efficacy and motivation. In this way the patient is empowered to manage their condition through patient-centred care.

Information-giving is essential to patient empowerment and effective self-care, and is thus an essential aspect of consultation skills. The nurse's demeanour and communication skills are perceived as inextricably linked to positive receipt of information. Although time consuming, an individualised approach to giving information is reported to improve patient concordance with medication (Timmins, 2007). Four key principles for giving information, which can be transferred to the general consultation, are to:

- Assess
- Plan
- Implement
- Evaluate.

Assess

Find out what the patient needs to know, and merge this with what you would like to address in this context. First, identify the patient's prior knowledge. If all the family are asthmatic, a parent might not require much information about the condition when their child is also diagnosed with the condition.

Ask the patient what would be helpful. This will vary between chronic disease, health advice to promote wound healing, and weight management. Responses to asking a patient what they would like to know vary. Some patients appreciate signposting to a particular resource but may not necessarily want the literature available in the surgery, while others are content with basic information. Some patients will be happy taking the tablets without further information.

Plan

Having identified the type of information the patient needs, or wants to know, it is time to plan how to deliver it. Choose which method to use: verbal, written, audio, a DVD, or maybe a mixture of methods? Use the method that is best for each individual's needs. Consider the patient's literacy and ethnicity. Are there leaflets available in other languages? What about audiotapes for the visually impaired patient? Also consider the family or carer. How much do they need or want to know? Involve the patient in the management plan to increase his commitment and adherence, and encourage him to accept some responsibility for his/her care (Silverman et al, 2005). Offer suggestions and advice, rather than instructions.

Implement

Most patients recall only 50–60% of the information given at a time (Silverman et al, 2005), and half of what they do recall is incorrect (Jackson and Skinner, 2007). It is therefore important not to bombard them with all they need to know in one session. One approach is to discuss the basics supported with literature, and develop this in following consultations. Reinforce information through repetition and summarising. This involves repetition of important points by the nurse, and re-statement of information by the patient. Sometimes it is helpful to use diagrams or visual aids to impart information. For example, this could be through showing pictures of normal and abnormal cervices to women when discussing a smear result, or using a diagram or model to explain how ear wax blocks the ear canal.

Look out for verbal or non-verbal cues indicating that the patient would like to ask a question, or appears confused by what has been said. Scenario 9 demonstrates the need for developing information over several weeks.

Scenario 9

Mrs B has been diagnosed with diabetes. The nurse assessed her existing knowledge of diabetes, which was very basic. She was aware that diabetes could lead to amputation. The nurse explained that diabetes was a complex condition, and that too much information would be confusing. They negotiated an education plan that would last for 6 weeks, covering different aspects of the condition each week. Mrs B asked permission to bring her husband to the sessions, because, in her words, 'I'm sure to forget something'. Each session was booked for 30 minutes, which allowed the nurse time to evaluate the amount of knowledge Mrs B retained from the previous week and led onto new information. The nurse supported her verbal information with leaflets from Diabetes UK. Gaps in knowledge were reinforced at each session and Mrs B was encouraged to ask questions. The programme was structured to include all aspects of lifestyle and social issues, including insurance, foot care, and managing minor illnesses.

Evaluate

Has the patient heard what has been said? How much can they recall? Ask them to repeat the advice they have been given to ensure they have understood the information and guidance which has been given to them.

It is recognised that many patients do not adhere to advice, even with the best supportive information. Silverman et al (2005) quote studies that report an average of 50% of patients do not adhere to medication regimes.

In each subsequent visit, whether for chronic disease management, weight management or contraception, it is essential that information is reiterated, rechecked with the patient and reinforced. Patients do forget, and they usually like to be reminded; *'Oh yes, I forgot about that'* is a common refrain. Refer to scenario 10.

Scenario 10

Nurse: 'Before you go, tell me what each inhaler does.'

Patient: 'The blue one is the one I have to take regularly, and the brown one when I can't breathe properly.'

Nurse: 'No, Mr A. I think I may have confused you. You take the brown one twice a day to keep your breathing tubes open, and the blue one when you're wheezy or short of breath.'

This approach places the blame on the information giver rather than the receiver, to reduce patient embarrassment.

Information giving must be given in chunks, jargon-free and reinforced. Consider the needs of each patient and respond appropriately. Negotiating a management plan is discussed further in Chapter 4.

Telephone consultations

Triaging, managing minor illness and follow up of chronic conditions can all be effectively achieved via the telephone, with patient satisfaction reported to be high (Silverman et al, 2005). There is little training for practice nurses in telephone interviewing, although many undertake an element of this in their daily work. Consultations may be no shorter than face-to-face ones, but play a useful role in minor illness, contraception and travel advice. It is important to remember that visual prompts and non-verbal gestures and signs are missing in telephone consultations. Nurses who undertake these consultations should have demonstrated their competency in undertaking consultations in routine care (RCN, 2006). *Box 2.9* lists the essential requirements for a successful telephone consultation.

It is impossible to hold a telephone consultation during the coffee break when the staff room is abuzz. If a receptionist wishes to transfer a call, either ask them to take the patient's telephone number to call later, or take the call in an empty office. This allows the nurse to access patient records and maintains patient confidentiality.

Box 2.9 Essential requirements for a successful
telephone consultation

- A conducive environment with minimal distractions and background noise
- Patient confidentiality and privacy throughout the consultation
- Access to patient records
- An empathetic manner, including reassurance and reiteration of the issues to confirm the caller's concern and needs
- Sufficient time to gain the necessary information to make a sound clinical decision
- The ability to provide clear and concise advice with guidance

(Source: RCN 2006)

Scenario 11

Miss P telephoned the surgery and asked to speak to a nurse about her pill. The nurses were busy, so she was informed that a nurse would phone her back as soon as one was free. The family planning trained nurse returned the call.

Nurse: 'Hello, this is Sister ... How can I help?'

Miss P: 'Oh, thank you getting back to me so soon. I've been really worried.'

Nurse: 'What's the problem?'

Miss P: 'I missed a pill last night and am not sure what to do.'

The nurse checks the patient records and clarifies that Miss P is taking the combined pill.

Nurse: 'How many pills are left in the packet?'

Miss P: 'Three.'

Nurse: 'Have you missed any other pills from this packet?

Miss P:'No.'

Nurse:'The advice is to take the last 3 pills but do not have a break before the next pack. Start the next packet straight away.' (repetition)

Miss P:'Oh, that's a relief. Thank you so much.'

Nurse:'Can you repeat what I've just said?'

Miss P:'Not to have a break but just carry on with my pill.' (ensures patient understands advice)

Nurse:'That's good. If you have any other concerns, don't hesitate to contact me.'

The nurse identified Miss P's concern and used her family planning expertise to reassure the patient and give appropriate advice. She used clear language and ensured the patient understood the advice. She then documented this advice in the patient notes (See Chapter 3 for more detail on documentation).

Information needs to be clear and simple, in chunks, and repeated to ensure patient understanding. Asking the patient to repeat an instruction is useful. Scenario 11 presents a common telephone consultation. This scenario can be adapted to advising on minor illnesses, such as flu symptoms or managing chicken pox.

All nurses will encounter difficult consultations on occasion. These include patients who are aggressive or manipulative, frequent or persistent callers, and those who have difficulty describing their problems. Nurses must only offer management advice on topics with which they are conversant, and consider their accountability at all times. Locally agreed protocols and guidelines would aid consistency in documenting telephone calls.

E-mail consultations

The legal concerns surrounding e-mail use in the medical field have been explored in the United States (Spiotta, 2003). Nurses frequently use e-mail for inter- and intra-professional communication, with the respondent replying at their convenience. However, there are advantages and disadvantages of this method of communication. See *Box 2.10*.

Box 2.10 Advantages and disadvantages of email consultations

Advantages
- The patient can deal with the nurse directly, and not through an intermediary
- The nurse can follow up a face to face consultation
- The patient can be referred to relevant sites on the Internet
- Email provides a hard copy of the consultation that does not occur with a telephone consultation.
- Email can reduce workload, as a query can be addressed at the end of a session, unless urgent
- It saves the patient taking time off work to see the nurse to ask a simple question.

Disadvantages
- Email cannot be used for urgent access to the nurse, as there is no guarantee that she will read the message in the necessary timeframe
- Email does not allow verbal and non-verbal signals to be transmitted
- Email can increase the workload
- Patients can abuse the system and bombard the nurse with questions
- Patient confidentiality may be compromised, as emails can go astray or sent to the wrong person by mistake.

(Source: Spiotta 2003)

Scenario 12

Mr and Mrs J and their three children attended for new patient health checks. The nurse asked for details of the children's vaccinations to record in the new records. Mrs J said she had these noted at home. The nurse suggested that Mrs J emailed her the details, which could then be transferred to the children's records. She received the data later that day, updated the records and deleted the email.

In scenario 12 this method of communication suited the parents who did not have to telephone the surgery (wait in a queue) and leave a message (which might have been misinterpreted or lost), and the nurse was able to complete her documentation. Mr and Mrs J did not consider the data confidential.

An email consultation is included within the legal framework for patient records, however you must consider the legal and practical aspects of email if considering this method of consultation.

Consultation skills with temporary patients

The practice population is transient, with a flow of patients to and from the practice list. This is more common in areas with student populations or travelling communities. The stages of consulting are no different to other patients, but the lack of prior knowledge of their health can create a challenge for negotiating an action plan.

A patient may present with a repeat prescription slip and a vague account of their medical history. Be patient and let the patient tell their story. If they have sufficient medication to last until their old notes arrive, be grateful. Do not try to guess for what conditions the medications have been prescribed. If possible, contact the patient's previous surgery to clarify medical history.

Managing the abusive or aggressive patient

It can be intimidating to be confronted by an angry, upset or frustrated patient. For simplicity the following text will use the word 'aggressive' to include angry, abusive and aggressive patients. Unfortunately there will always be the occasional patient who will express anger or become aggressive in the surgery. This might be because they had been kept waiting, are very anxious, or are generally difficult. There are many factors that can predispose a patient to display aggressive behaviour (see *Box 2.11*). The skill is to defuse the aggression and continue the consultation safely.

It is recognised that aggression in the workplace can lead to emotional upset and anxiety (Flores, 2008). Be conversant with the practice policy on managing aggression. If there isn't a policy, liaise with the practice team to compile one. The consulting room should be fitted with an alarm system with which to summon assistance when required. Again, if this is not available, discuss this with the practice manager as part of the health and safety policy. Personal safety is paramount as it can be difficult to know which patient will become aggressive, and the consulting room should be arranged to allow the nurse to exit the room ahead of the patient (see Chapter 1). Arrange the room so the nurse's chair is nearest the door wherever possible. Although they are not responsible for the actions or omissions in the reception and waiting areas, nurses should be alert to a patient's aggression through their body language and verbal outbursts.

Box 2.11 Factors predisposing to aggression

The patient
- Being under the influence of alcohol or drugs
- Hypoglycaemia, acute febrile illness
- History of violence
- Social isolation
- Psychological disorders such as bipolar disease or schizophrenia

At reception or in the waiting area
- Not being given an appointment
- Being overheard by others
- Long waiting time to speak to someone
- Noisy children running about
- Too hot or too cold
- Uncomfortable seating

In the consulting room
- Nurse running behind with appointments and keeping patient waiting
- Already wound up from waiting room experience
- Inappropriate use of humour
- Nurse attending to computer rather than patient
- Nurse busy, under pressure
- Nurse inflicts pain during a procedure

(adapted from More 2009; Flores 2008)

Efforts to de-escalate/defuse a difficult situation might be achieved through:

- (A) Removing the trigger from the patient
- (B) Active listening
- (C) Addressing the problem and discussing a solution
- (D) Appearing calm, interested but assertive.

It would be expedient to address the cause of the patient's aggression before it escalates, even if the patient is not due to see that particular professional. The following scenario is all too common in general practice.

Scenario 13

It is Monday morning. The nurse goes into the waiting room to collect her next patient. Mr S is shouting at the receptionist at the front desk. The waiting room is full. What would you do?

Options:

Collect your patient and scuttle back to your room, hoping no-one saw you
Divert to the practice manager's office to alert her to the incident
Walk calmly up to Mr S and ask him whether you can help

All options are reasonable. However, option 3 could be regarded as the most professional approach to take. Patients are often aggressive to the ancillary staff, but respond in a different manner to a nurse. The consultation might carry on as follows:

Nurse [quietly]: 'Good morning, Mr S. There seems to be a problem here. Would you like to come into my office and talk about it?'

Mr S [in a raised voice]: 'I'm trying to get a prescription and they're not helping' [pointing to the receptionist]

Nurse: 'Let's try and sort this out. Would you like to come with me?'

Nurse apologises to her waiting patient and reassures her that she will not be long, but to re-book if she wishes. Mr S follows the nurse into the consulting room.

Nurse: 'Now, Mr S. Could you explain what the problem is?'

Mr S: 'I've run out of tablets and can't get any more. The receptionist said there isn't an appointment until tonight. I need to take my tablets this morning.' [brandishes repeat prescription slip]

In this scenario the nurse has demonstrated all her consultation skills while defusing the situation. She removed Mr S from the trigger (A), took him to a quiet place, listened to his side of the story (B), and identified and dealt with the problem (C), and remained calm throughout (D). Although the next patient was slightly delayed, the atmosphere in the waiting room returned to normal. The next patient had been advised that her appointment would be slightly delayed, but preferred this to re-booking. Although it could be argued that Mr S should wait for an appointment, the reception staff do not always have the authority or confidence to deal with these situations. Anecdotally, the patient is usually humble with the nurse whilst aggressive at the desk. Also, dealing with the situation as soon as possible reduces the anxiety of waiting patients. It is important to note that the nurse could have asked for a chaperone for this consultation if there was a risk of physical violence.

Aggressive behaviour typically escalates in three stages: anxiety, verbal aggression, and physical aggression (Flores, 2008). Identifying and managing a patient in the anxiety stage can prevent escalation to stages two and three. More (2009) and Miles (2008) offer a list of 'do's' and 'do not's' of anger management that are relevant to dealing with aggression (*Box 2.12*).

Scenario 14 considers the management of a patient who became aggressive when given appropriate advice for diabetic management.

Box 2.12 Do's and do not's of anger management

Do

- Remember it is the patient and not you who are angry
- Look at the patient, listen and hear him out
- Give the patient attention, understanding and sympathy
- Use non-verbal body language to show attention
- Take any threat of violence seriously
- Have an escape route ready
- Leave an escape route for the patient
- Keep on your guard until the incident is over
- Avoid putting yourself in a vulnerable position
- Call for help if you feel physically threatened.

Do not

- Contradict the patient
- Behave in a combative or threatening way
- Take personal offence at anything that is said to you
- Interrupt the patient in the middle of an outburst
- Caution the patient's choice of words
- Make promises you cannot keep

(Source: More 2009, Miles 2008)

Scenario 14

Mr D was a 70-year-old man with a history of Type 2 diabetes. He had attended for routine blood tests prior to his regular diabetic review. Two weeks later he saw Nurse A to review the results and discuss his next action plan. The HbA1c was raised, indicating poor glycaemic control. After ascertaining that Mr D had no apparent infection or new medications that might have influenced the HbA1c, Nurse A explained the blood results and followed the practice protocol for diabetes management, looking at lifestyle change to reduce the blood sugars. Mr D became angry and accused Nurse A of harassment. He then filed a formal complaint and refused to attend any further diabetic clinic appointments. Mr D saw a doctor for all future reviews.

Why did this happen?

Mr D did not accept the suggested action plan to help reduce the blood sugars to target levels. He maintained that Nurse A did not know what she was talking about.

The NMC Code states that nurses must act in the patient's best interests (NMC, 2008). Nurse A was patient, explained the blood results and how raised blood sugars damage the body. She followed a standard protocol to ensure Mr D received the best advice. In hindsight Nurse A could have terminated the consultation as soon as Mr D became angry and referred him to the doctor for advice.

When dealing with an angry patient, maintain non-threatening eye contact, and try not to adopt an aggressive stance. Break off eye contact when you speak to demonstrate a wish to be conciliatory. Consider personal safety at all times. Do not go alone in to a room with an aggressive patient. Stay at least four feet away from the patient if you anticipate a violent outburst. If there is a real threat of violence, move away and press the panic button (Tate, 2003). Anger and aggression can lead to personality clashes that subsequently result in a barrier to the consultation. Where abuse or violence has occurred it is essential to complete a clinical incident report. This documentation is evidence that can be used to improve the work environment and staff and patient safety.

Potential barriers within the consultation

No matter how much preparation goes into a consultation, or how experienced the nurse is, there will always be occasions when there is a barrier between the nurse and patient. This section will offer suggestions on how to overcome some of the common barriers, listed in *Box 2.13*.

Box 2.13 Barriers to communication

- Cultural (language, ethnic, religion and social differences)
- Linguistic (different language or vocabulary)
- Checking the clock or watch
- Turning away from the patient to read or write notes
- Not allowing the patient to complete their story
- The use of closed or leading questions
- Being over familiar
- Body language
- Proximity – closeness – distance
- Patient's health beliefs
- Lack of time
- Assumptions or prejudices
- Environment
- Interruptions
- Personality clashes

Culture
It is important to respect an individual's culture, whether this relates to having a female chaperone, avoiding eye contact, or managing dietary advice within Ramadan.

Linguistic
Difficulties with language can clearly have an impact when obtaining consent for treatment. The use of interpreters is discussed in Chapter 9. Many patients cannot understand technical language — they do not understand about microvascular and macrovascular damage in diabetes, but do understand the words 'kidney damage' and 'blindness'. The expression '*Please wee in this pot*' might be more appropriate than '*Please do an MSU*'.

Checking the clock or watch
Checking the clock or watch suggests you are either bored, or very busy.

If it is the latter, be honest and state that there are several patients waiting and bring the consultation to a close. Ask the patient to make another appointment if necessary.

Turning away from patients to read or write notes

Turning away to read or write notes removes the eye contact and rapport that occurred on greeting the patient. Read the patient notes before calling them. Try to position the computer at an angle so the patient and screen can be seen. If there is need to turn away, apologise and say: *'I'm sorry to have my back to you, but I just want to check your records'*.

Not allowing the patient to complete their story

The patient will understandably feel ignored if they cannot finish telling their story. Listen to them and do not interrupt to ask questions, but wait until the patient has finishing speaking.

The use of closed or leading questions

As mentioned previously closed and leading questions do not allow the patient the opportunity to elaborate their concerns. The consultation may appear short and sharp, so include open questions where appropriate.

Being over-familiar

Over familiarity is a two-way barrier. The patient wants a professional consultation, while the nurse wishes to be friendly, approachable but remain professional. The nurse who touches the patient in sympathy might be seen as over-familiar. This can be a difficult balance to achieve at times. Over familiarity from the patient may make the nurse defensive and wish to conclude the consultation as soon as possible, which is not in the patient's best interests. Be honest and and tell the patient that certain behaviour is unacceptable.

Body language

The importance of body language has already been discussed. Again, this is a two-way barrier. The nurse must learn to express positive body language as well as recognising negative signs from the patient.

Proximity: closeness–distance

How close is closeness and how far is distance? Personal space is important. The patient who leans forward and is almost touching the nurse can appear threatening. The nurse who talks to the patient from the other side of the room can appear distant. The skill is to reach a happy medium, where nurse and patient are comfortable.

Patient's health beliefs

A barrier is created when dealing with the patient whose health beliefs do not fit the norm. For example, Mr G's father smoked and drank all his life and he lived to be 101, so he is not going to change his lifestyle. In these instances it is safer to offer support when he wishes it, rather than give him information that he does not want.

Lack of time

The provision of psychological care can be time consuming (Towers, 2007), but so can undertaking complex wound care, or counselling about a chronic disease. Spending time talking to patients can be viewed as time wasting, especially as the end result is not quantifiable. Scenario 15 gives an example of combining physical and psychological care in one appointment.

Assumptions and prejudices

Assumptions and prejudices are common. For example, the nurse might assume that the female patient who attends wearing traditional Muslim dress

---

Scenario 15

The nurse had checked the patient records before calling Mrs C and was aware that the patient was attending for a postoperative dressing following bowel surgery. Mrs C entered the room, sat down and was visibly distressed. It transpired that the surgeon was unable to remove the cancer and no further treatment was available. The nurse continued with the dressing, allowing Mrs C to share her feelings. The consultation overran by 10 minutes.

Why did it happen?
Mrs C had attended the outpatient clinic the previous day and been given the news that no further treatment was possible. She had no family with whom to discuss her fears.

What could have happened?
If the nurse had not allowed Mrs C to share her anxieties, the stress might be detrimental to her wound healing and psychological wellbeing. The added anxiety could affect her sleep, which could lead to the need for medication.

Reflection
The extra time spent enable Mrs C to unburden her anxiety, and she left the surgery knowing she could discuss these worries at future appointments. Future appointments were booked as double slots to prevent reoccurrence of this situation.

---

cannot speak English, whereas in fact, she is second generation and has excellent English. Prejudice against minority groups of all types can be a major barrier (see Chapter 9).

In another example, the patient with poor personal hygiene is likely to receive a short consultation as the nurse rushes to open the windows. There is no easy answer to this latter barrier, except take a deep breath, or breathe very gently.

Environment

The importance of a welcoming environment was discussed in Chapter 1. Try to position the furniture to reduce the you-and-me barrier. Ensure privacy and confidentiality.

Interruptions

Any interruption can create a barrier within a consultation. This could be a colleague seeking a piece of equipment, a telephone call or an emergency. The following scenario is a common experience in some practices and can be disruptive to the consultation.

Scenario 16

The nurse was discussing the self-management of chronic obstructive airways disease with Mr D. She had explained how to use the oral steroids and antibiotics, and had printed a personalised self-management plan. The nurse was just about to reinforce the points to the patient when the doctor then rang the nurse requesting a chaperone.

Options:

1. Acknowledge a chaperone is required and tell the doctor that you will come at the end of your present consultation
2. Leave Mr D and attend to the doctor's request.
3. Ask a colleague to chaperone in your place.

The telephone call was a distraction for both the nurse and patient. The nurse was aware that the doctor was on call and had a busy surgery, so she wanted to support him. In this situation, the consultation was almost over, so the nurse chose option 1, which allowed the consultation to continue with minimal distraction. Option 2 could have resulted in Mr D becoming confused about his self-management plan.

Personality clashes

There will always be occasions when the patient and nurse do not gain the necessary rapport for a satisfactory consultation. This may not be anyone's fault, but simply human nature. In these instances it is sensible to rebook the patient with a colleague or doctor to avoid confrontation. A patient who does not accept the advice being given might wish to see another professional in the hope that they will give the advice the patient wants to hear (for example refer to scenario 14). However, hopefully doctors and nurses do give the same advice to ensure equity of care.

Barriers relating to consulting skills with children and adolescents, and minority groups are discussed in the relevant chapters.

Summary

Effective communication also has positive outcomes for nurses. It is gratifying to hear patient satisfaction following a consultation. Listen to what the patient has to say. Let them tell their story. Ensure they have understood any instructions, whether about medication regimes, self-management or future appointments. Use both verbal and non-verbal communication to gain a rapport with the patient and maximise each consultation. Reduce potential barriers by planning and adapting consultation skills where necessary.

Key points

- Communication skills are the key to a successful consultation
- Consider body language
- Develop good listening skills
- Remove potential barriers

Edwards M (2008) *The Informed Practice Nurse*. 2nd edn. Wiley, Chichester

Flores N (2008) Dealing with an angry patient. *Nursing 2007* **38**(5): 30–1

Hornsten A, Lundman B, Selstan E, Sandstrom H (2005) Patient satisfaction with diabetes care. *Journal of Advanced Nursing* **51**(6): 609–17

Kaufman G (2008) Patient assessment: effective consultation and history taking. *Nursing Standard* **23**(4): 50–6

Jackson M, Skinner J (2007) Improving consultations in general practice for Somali patients: a qualitative study. *Diversity in Health and Social Care* **4**(1): 61–7

Miles J (2008) Effective communication. *Practice Nurse* **35**(2): 42–7

Mind Tools (2008) *Improve listening skills with Mind Tools*. www.mindtools.com accessed 20/10/2008

More W (2009) *Managing Aggression and Violence. A model for general practices and good safety habits for staff.* www.scot.nhs.uk/.../AggressOptions.htm

accessed 2/3/2009

Nursing and Midwifery Council (2008) *The Code. Standards of conduct, performance and ethics for nurses and midwives.* NMC, London

Prentice P (2008) How practice nurse and patients can help each other. BMJ Learning. Practice Nurse CPD. http://learning.bmj.com accessed 21/1/2008

Richards S, Gregory S (2005) Developing consultation skills. *Practice Nurse* **29**(11): 13–20

Robertson K (2008) The importance of communication skills. Practice nurse CPD. BMJ Learning. http://learning.bmj.com accessed 20/10/08

Royal College of Nursing (2006) *Telephone advice lines for people with long term conditions. Guidance for nursing practitioners.* RCN, London

Silverman J, Kurtz S, Draper J (2005) *Skills for Communicating with Patients.* 2nd edn. Radcliffe Publishing, Oxford

Spiotta VL (2003) JONA'S Legal Concerns Surrounding E-mail Use in a Medical Practice. *Healthcare, Law, Ethics and Regulation* **5**(3): 53–7

Tate P (2003) *The Doctor's Communication Handbook.* 4th edn. Radcliffe Medical Press Ltd, Oxford

Timmins F (2007) Communication skills: information giving. *Nurse prescribing* **5**(10): 437–41

Towers R (2007) Providing psychological support for patients with cancer. *Nursing Standard* **22**(12): 50–7

CHAPTER 3

Ethical issues

The principles of ethics are integral to all patient consultations, including confidentiality and consent with reference to the Data Protection Act 1998. This chapter aims to provide the reader with an insight into some of the issues that may be encountered during any consultation. For further information, please refer to texts on ethics. Issues relating specifically to children are discussed in detail in Chapter 5.

Confidentiality

Confidentiality is one of the most important issues to consider during a patient consultation. The patient would lose all confidence in the health system if he thought his confidentiality was being breached. The NMC Code (2008) states that:

- You must respect people's right to confidentiality
- You must ensure people are informed about how and why information is shared by those who will be providing their care
- You must disclose information if you believe someone may be at risk of harm in line with the law of the country in which you are practising.

Sometimes a patient will share personal information that they do not want recorded or passed to a third person. They have a right to expect that their wishes will be complied with, for if they cannot rely on confidentiality they will be unlikely to seek help when they desperately need it. However, it could be detrimental to patient care if relevant data is omitted from a patient's records. Scenario 1 overleaf highlights the potential problems faced by nurses.

Information should be shared on a who needs to know basis only. It is impractical to gain consent every time information is shared within the team. The nurse must gain consent to share information, but patients rarely refuse when their best interests are being served.

Scenario 1

Mrs C was seeing the nurse every 2 weeks for weight management support. She stated she was following the recommended lifestyle advice and was losing weight at 0.5-1kg at each visit. She did not attend for several weeks, but responded to a telephone call to enquire about her progress and continue motivation. Mrs C attended and was re-weighed, and was noted to have gained weight. The consultation went:

Mrs C: 'I'm back on track now.'

Nurse: 'What does that mean?' (open question)

Mrs C: 'I've stopped chocolate' (body language suggests she has something else to share)

Nurse: 'Would you like to talk about this?' (offers the opportunity to share)

Mrs C [nods and looks ashamed]: 'I've had a problem for some years but never talked about it. My husband has just found out. I have phases, but I'm over it now.' (shares history of bulimia)

Mrs C: 'Please don't put this in my notes.'

The nurse understood that Mrs C was ashamed about her eating disorder and respected her wishes. She discussed the risk of bulimia, discussed oral care to prevent dental caries, and arranged a follow-up appointment. If the situation deteriorated or Mrs C suffered ill health, she would then advise the patient that she would have to share this information with the doctor. Did she make the right decision? What would you have done?

In the situation described in scenario 2 the nurse had to share the information with the doctor for an effective consultation, but ensured she had patient consent to share personal details.

There are, however, instances when acting in the interest of the patient may conflict with the interest of society, for example when the patient is alcoholic and continues to drive (refer to scenario 3). The nurse has a responsibility to report this to her employer, who may then report this to the DVLA.

Scenario 2

Dave is homosexual, but is not open about his sexuality. He was booked in with the nurse who had seen him for his new patient health check.

Nurse: 'Hello, Dave. How are you? What can I do for you today?' (open question)

Dave [appears anxious]: 'I went to a party last weekend and I don't know what happened.'

Nurse: 'How do you mean?' (allows elaboration)

Dave: 'I woke up and found my pants across the room, [looks more anxious] I don't do that sort of thing, [implies anal sex], I'm frantic. My bum is sore.'

Nurse: 'Would you prefer to discuss this with a doctor?'

Dave: 'No. I know you and that's why I've come to see you. Will you have a look?' [patient has rapport with the nurse]

Nurse locks the door, guides Dave to the couch, draws the curtains, and asks him to lower his trousers and pants, and lie on the couch in a lateral position with knees bent. On examination the anal region is inflamed, with a slight discharge.

Nurse: 'I really think you should see the doctor. If it's all right I'll explain the situation to him, to save you having to go over it again. Is that OK?' (gains consent to share information)

Dave [reluctantly]: 'Yes. I suppose so. OK then.'

The nurse sought the senior partner and explained the history. The doctor entered the room, was sensitive in his examination, took a swab and explained to Dave that he should go to the genito-urinary medicine clinic, as he may have a sexually transmitted infection (STI).

The doctor left the nurse to explain that Dave should have a full screen, as he was at risk of a range of STI's. She gave him a card with the clinic contact number and encouraged him to attend as soon as possible. The swab was positive to gonorrhoea. The patient left the practice so there was no follow up.

Scenario 3

Mr G was alcoholic. He drank 120 units of alcohol a week, but still worked. He had to drive with his work. The doctor had noted on the patient records that Mr G had been advised to contact the DLVA as he should not be driving. During a consultation for venepuncture, the nurse discovered that Mr G had not followed the doctor's advice, was still drinking and still driving, thus putting other drivers, passengers and pedestrians at risk.

Options:

1. Tell the patient she would have to notify the DVLA herself
2. Tell the patient that she would have to inform the doctor, who would then notify the DVLA
3. Ignore the situation, as it wasn't her problem.

In this instance the nurse chose option 2. She devolved the problem to a higher authority. Option 3 would have breached the NMC Code.

Careless talk

Confidential information can be inadvertently released into the public domain when discussing a patient's problems with a colleague in a public place, such as in an office that is open to a waiting area, or on a telephone in reception. This can cause complete loss of faith in the health service. Confidential details may be passed around over coffee so that information that a patient shared in confidence with one professional becomes public property.

It is essential that nurses consider the issue of confidentiality in all consultations, whether face-to-face, or telephone. Only divulge information with the patient's express consent, unless there is a good reason.

Consent

It is a basic rule of law that no one has any right to touch another person without their consent. Therefore a nurse may not do anything to a patient without first gaining their agreement, ensuring that the patient understands and agrees to the treatment suggested. Consent must not be coerced and the benefit of any intervention must outweigh any harmful effects.
The NMC Code (2008) states that:

'You must ensure that you gain consent before you begin any treatment or care.'

Exceptions to this law involve some aspects of nursing care. This exception also permits the nurse to care for unconscious patients, which may be a simple faint or the need for cardio-pulmonary resuscitation in primary care (Edwards, 2008).

Informed consent

Informed consent has been defined as the patient's right to know what is entailed before any procedure is carried out (Chadwick and Tadd, 1992). The nurse must ensure that the patient is fully informed about any procedure or treatment that she is going to undertake in order for consent to be obtained, even when they have given implied consent by attending the surgery. The patient must be competent to understand and decide voluntarily, having been given accurate information which they can understand to authorize the agreed plan of care.

It has been argued that informed consent does not exist genuinely between professional and patient, as the patient can never fully understand the information they are given (Beauchamp and Childress, 2001). This reinforces the issue of an unequal contract between the health professional and patient. It may be appropriate in some instances to defer a procedure or treatment until informed consent can be obtained, as stress and illness may influence the patient's ability to make a rational decision.

Scenario 4 relates to coercion in practice. In this instance the nurse should be comfortable accepting the patient's decision, even though it would be in his best interests to have the injection. If the patient had been coerced into having the injection and suffered unpleasant side effects, he would lose trust in the nurse. Meeting targets should not take precedence over patient choice.

Implied consent

Nurses working within general practice will usually encounter implied consent. It would be assumed that a patient who voluntarily attends a flu clinic and proffers an arm for vaccination has given implied consent to the procedure. However, women may be sent to the nurse by the doctor for vaginal swabs without understanding, for example, the implication of a positive chlamydia result. A woman may be shocked when counselled

---

Scenario 4

It is October. The fridge is full of flu vaccine. There are targets to meet. Mr A appears at the nurse's door, having been sent by the doctor. The nurse ascertains that Mr A has been sent for a flu jab because he has coronary heart disease. He has never had the injection before and does not want it now. He only came because the doctor sent him.

Options:

1. Disregard his indecision and give the injection before he can think about it
2. Discuss the advantages and disadvantages of the vaccine and allow Mr A to make a decision.
3. Accept that Mr A does not want the injection but feels pressurised by the doctor. Suggest he comes back if he changes his mind.

Option 1 would be classed as coercion. Mr A does not want the flu jab but has been sent to the nurse anyway. It could be argued that he could easily have gone home and ignored the doctor's 'suggestion'. Patients often feel they must do what the doctor says, even when they do not want to. Options 2 and 3 allow the patient to make his own choice, which the nurse should respect.

---

and informed that chlamydia is a sexually transmitted infection, and if positive the woman would be advised to attend the genitourinary clinic. It is important to ensure that the patient is fully aware of the implications of any investigation before it is taken. Scenario 5 relates to venepuncture.

Consent is also discussed in the chapters relating to children, disability and cultural diversity.

Advocacy

Advocacy in healthcare involves speaking up for, or acting on behalf of, a patient, self or colleague. This is especially important where a person is at risk of being excluded, ignored or mistreated. It is also making sure that people are fully involved in the decisions that affect their lives, and that their views are taken into account (Partners in Advocacy, 2007). Within the context of consultation skills, this will be related to the patient. Advocacy can help patients to:

Scenario 5

The doctor has asked the nurse to squeeze Mr B into her surgery list for venepuncture as it 'will only take a minute', and will save him having to ask a family member to bring him back. Mr B enters the room, sits down and proffers his arm. He has given implied consent to the procedure.

Options:

1. The nurse takes the blood and Mr B leaves the room
2. The nurse explains what the tests are for, what the results might mean and ensures Mr B knows how to access the results. She also ensures he knows if and when the doctor wishes to review him.

Option 1 is quick and easy. A simple task fitted in between patients for Mr B's convenience. Option 2 does not 'only take a minute', but is important to ensure that Mr B is aware of the implications of the blood test, which is to check the prostate specific antigen (PSA). The nurse chose option 2. It transpired that Mr B had a raised PSA, which led to further invasive investigations, for which he was prepared.

In an ideal world the doctor would explain why he is asking for the blood tests and what the results imply, but unfortunately this is not always the case. The nurse who initiates or undertakes any investigations during her consultations should ensure the patient is fully aware of the follow up process and implications of the results (NMC, 2008).

- Make clear their own views and wishes
- Express and present their views effectively and faithfully
- Obtain independent advice and accurate information
- Negotiate and resolve conflict.

As an advocate for autonomy, the nurse assists the patient to make an authentic decision that meets his/her own values and lifestyle. There may be occasions during a consultation where the nurse must consider whether the patient requires her to be an advocate, or whether it is more appropriate to involve an outside advocacy source. The nurse may also act as the patient's advocate if decisions made by others conflict with the person's wishes. A simple example is when the patient requires treatment for hypertension but the patient wishes to continue non-pharmacological measures for a longer period before embarking on medication. The patient is scared to refuse the treatment in case the doctor is annoyed. The nurse acts as advocate by speaking up for the patient to the doctor, explaining her views and gaining the doctor's approval for the management plan.

If a nurse is unable to act on a patient's behalf she should refer him to a local independent advocacy scheme. Each Primary Care Trust (PCT) has a Patient Advocacy Liaison Service (PALS) to which the patient can be referred, and who will act for the patient. See scenario 6.

Scenario 6

Mrs B presents for a dressing for a laceration to her shin. The nurse cleaned and dressed the wound and arranged a follow-up appointment. Whilst documenting her actions, she noted that Mrs B had been referred to the eye infirmary 12 months previously for cataracts. The consultation went:

Nurse: 'How did you get on at the eye infirmary?'

Mrs B: 'I'm on the waiting list for surgery.'

Nurse: 'When are you due to have the operation?'

Mrs B: 'They keep changing the date. I've been put back three times so far. They say there's no money. I'm waiting for another appointment.'

Options:

1. The nurse contacts the eye infirmary to try to expedite the appointment (takes valuable nurse time)
2. The nurse asks the doctor to contact the surgeon (too busy)
3. The nurse offers the patient details of the local PALS to work on her behalf (patient takes some responsibility).

The nurse chose option 3. When seen for the next dressing review, Mrs B was delighted to report that her appointment date was for 2 weeks time.

Patient autonomy

Definition of autonomy

Autonomy is derived from the Greek *autos* ('self') and *nomos* ('rule', 'governance' or 'law') (Beauchamp and Childress, 2001).

An autonomous person has the ability to be able to choose for himself and is said to be self-determining. Healthcare professionals have a moral obligation to give patients as much unbiased information as possible to make informed autonomous decisions. It is not possible for someone to make a decision of their own free will if they do not know the options open to them.

Scenario 7

Mr S is a 58-year-old teacher who attends for hypertension monitoring, having had two previously high readings. The nurse advised him on the last occasion that medication would be an option if the blood pressure remained raised. Non-pharmacological measures have already been discussed and implemented. His blood pressure today is 160/100. Although he admits that stress at work may be contributory, Mr S is keen to have treatment as his father had a cardiovascular event aged 65 years old. The nurse is an independent prescriber and discusses the medication options. The practice follows the British Hypertension Guidelines, but she still explains the side effects of different types of medication.

Options:

1. Thiazide: increased diuresis, gout
2. Angiotensin converting enzyme (ACE) inhibitor: annoying cough
3. Betablocker: cold extremities, lethargy, impotence
4. Calcium channel blocker: flushing, headache

Mr S agrees to try an ACE inhibitor. On review he admits to a slight cough, but is willing to continue as his blood pressure is now to target.

In scenario 7 Mr S was involved in his care, was aware of the options and potential side effects of the medication. Encouraging autonomy is time consuming but can result in improved treatment concordance that may save further surgery appointments and/or reduce patient morbidity (Edwards, 2008).

Trainees present during consultations

Many general practices offer training facilities so a patient may find a student nurse, family planning student, medical student or GP registrar present during the consultation. Written consent should be obtained before the consultation to give patients the opportunity to decline the observer if they so wish before they are confronted with the learner. This is particularly relevant for intimate consultations such as cervical cytology, when the woman may prefer not to have either a male or female learner in attendance. Even if there is no objection it is important that the patient is allowed to control the flow of information.

Although the NMC Code (2008) states that: '*You must facilitate students and others to develop their confidence*' and '*You must be willing to share your skills and experience for the benefit of your colleagues*' the requirements of the student must not take precedence over the need to seek consent.

From experience many patients enjoy having trainees present, as they learn more about their condition during the consultations. Some women are happy to have a trainee present for a pre-smear consultation but request they are not present during the procedure. Others are more than happy for a trainee to observe or practice. The nurse should not make assumptions about a patient's preferences.

Documentation

Accurate documentation is an essential component of all consultations (NMC, 2008). Good record keeping helps protect the welfare of patients (NMC, 2007) (see *Box 3.1*).

Patient concerns, all findings, advice given and any agreed action plan should be recorded as soon as possible after a consultation. Do not wait until the end of surgery to complete patient records as important details might be omitted in error. However, do make a note of any referrals that require action, and deal with these at the end of surgery. Documentation must

---

Box 3.1 Record keeping

Good record keeping promotes:
- High standards of clinical care
- Continuity of care
- Better communication and dissemination of information between members of the practice team
- An accurate account of treatment and care planning and delivery
- The ability to identify risk and detect problems, such as changes in the patient's condition at an early stage
- The concept of confidentiality.

(Source: NMC, 2007)

---

be clearly written, factual, consistent and accurate. It should not include abbreviations, jargon, meaningless phrases, irrelevant speculation, and must be objective and not subjective: 'Smell of alcohol on breath' is objective, whilst 'appears drunk' is subjective. Wherever possible the record should be recorded with the patient or carer involvement and recorded in terms that the patient can understand.

In scenario 8 it would be reasonable to document that Mr P was unreceptive to health advice at the present time and future support was offered.

Scenario 8

Mr P was sent to see the nurse for weight management. The nurse welcomed him and invited him to sit down. His body language suggested that he was not pleased to be in the room. The nurse could not gain eye contact as Mr P sat with crossed legs and gazed at the wall behind her. The consultation progressed:

Nurse: 'How can I help you today?'

Mr P: 'The doctor sent me to see you about losing weight.'

Nurse: 'And how do you feel about this?'

Mr : 'Hmm. I don't know what the fuss is about. I'm OK'. [Deep sigh, gazes at wall].

Nurse: 'Would you like help to lose weight?'

Mr P: 'Not really.'

Nurse: 'Well, I can't help you now, but I'm here to support you when you feel ready.'

Scenario 9 and 10 overleaf highlights the importance of clear record keeping. The nurse in this case had used best practice to assess the wound, made the decision that it required the expertise of a hand surgeon, and made the appropriate referral. Although Dan chose not to attend, the nurses continued to offer him non-judgemental nursing care until the wound healed. Subsequent nerve damage was unfortunate but no blame could be attached to the nurse.

Scenario 9

Dan is 17-years-old. He was an emergency walk-in consultation at 12.00 hours, having had a laceration to his right hand. The nurse took a history, examined the hand and made a judgment that the wound was too deep to suture in the surgery and required the skills of the hand clinic in secondary care. She dressed the wound to prevent infection, and advised him to attend A&E. She documented the treatment and advice in the patient notes. These read:

'Laceration to right palm at base of thumb 1 hour ago. Wound 3cm long, subcutaneous fat visible. Not suitable for suturing in practice. Advised to attend casualty to assess for nerve damage. Pressure bandage and sling applied.'

Dan presented the following day for a dressing, having chosen not to attend the hospital. The wound was uncovered. It was too late to suture the wound, which was now inflamed and showing signs of infection.

Dan attended the surgery for follow-up dressings and the wound subsequently healed after several weeks. However Dan was left with nerve damage to his fingers.

Implications for practice
Dan required the expertise of secondary care to assess and manage his injury and preserve nerve function.

The contemporaneous patient records were evidence that Dan had been advised to attend hospital. Therefore a patient complaint due to the delayed healing or nerve damage would not be upheld in a court of law.

Telephone advice

All telephone calls made or received relating to patient care should be documented in the patient records. This might read:

'Telephone call from patient — late for Depo Provera. Episode of unprotected sexual intercourse last night. Appointment booked with nurse this afternoon to discuss emergency contraception.'

This information clearly states that the patient has a booked appointment. If she fails to attend and subsequently attends with an unwanted pregnancy, the nurse has evidence to prove she acted in the patient's best interests by offering to see her the same day.

Scenario 10

Mrs E attends for her hypertension review. She has 'white coat syndrome', and her blood pressure is always high when taken in the surgery. Mrs E states that her blood pressure is always lower on her home readings. What do you do?

Options:

1. Always document the surgery reading
2. Always document the patient's home readings
3. Ask Mrs E to bring her machine to surgery, with the home readings, and compare the 2 sphygmomanometers to assess the accuracy of Mrs E's machine.

Option 1 may lead to over treatment of the hypertension. Option 2 may lead to under treatment, if the machine is not accurate. Option 3 allows comparison of readings. If the machines give the same raised blood pressure in surgery, it would be reasonable to accept the home readings and document these in the patient records. Always state where the blood pressure has been recorded, either at home or in the surgery. This is also important when the patient attends with blood pressure readings taken at another source, such as an outpatient appointment or the pharmacy.

Liaison with the wider primary health care team

Clear and accurate documentation is also pertinent when the nurse discusses a patient with a medical or nursing colleague and an action plan is agreed. For example, when a wound care specialist has been contacted for advice about wound management, the patient's record might read:

'Seen by wound care nurse X. Wound to be dressed three times a week. Potassium permanganate soaks to be applied and left on the wound for 15 minutes. Remove, apply flamazine cream to area, cover with absorbent pad. To be reviewed by X in 2 weeks.'

The regime is clearly documented for all staff to understand and follow, ensuring continuity of care.

'While I am here'

Many patients have an afterthought following their consultation. They start to rise out of their seat to leave then say: '*While I am here, nurse…*'. If dealt with before completing the documentation from the first problem, there is a danger that errors will occur. Smith (2009) suggests making a note of the first details, or saying: '*One moment please. I just need to finish typing up this note first*'. Alternatively, ask the patient to make another appointment to discuss the problem.

Patient records are sometimes called as evidence when a patient makes a complaint, either in criminal or professional proceedings. If you have completed accurate records that detail your assessment, what you advised or care given, and any referrals made to senior staff, you have proof of safe professional practice. It is recognised that '*…if it is not recorded it has not been done*' (NMC 2007).

Patient/parent-held records

Shared care records are commonly used in warfarin monitoring, arthritis and antenatal care and for child records. Patient-held records involve the patient sharing in, and having ownership of, his own record, be more closely involved in their own care, and improve multidisciplinary communication. The patient or parent should be informed of the purpose and importance of the record, and their responsibility for keeping it safe (NMC, 2007). The importance of accurate child health records is highlighted in scenario 11.

In this scenario the nurse checked all available documentation. The injections were clearly entered and dated in the child health record (the red book). The nurse was open with Mrs M and explained that this was a human error, reassuring her that no further injections were needed and that Josh's records were now correct. If she had not asked to see the red book, Josh would have received unnecessary immunisations. The nurse was accountable for her actions, and could have been deemed negligent for not checking all records.

The patient must be a partner in this, controlling the flow of information and not just transporting the record. Ensure that relevant data is added at every consultation to promote continuity of care.

Data Protection Act

The Data Protection Act 1998 covers confidentiality of patient information

---

Scenario 11

Mrs M has brought Josh for his pre school booster. He is on the immunisation sheet for his MMR and diphtheria, tetanus whooping cough, polio and hib. The nurse checks the computer record. The immunisations have not been given.

Nurse: 'Have you got Josh's red book with you?'

Mrs M: 'Oh yes.' [Delves in bag and retrieves red book.]

Nurse looks at the immunisation record page.

Nurse: 'Oh. Josh had this last year. He doesn't need another injection. I'm sorry, but there has been a mistake somewhere along the line. I'll just put this on his records.'

---

including medical records. It includes aspects of collecting, processing, storing and transferring data. Nurses have a legal as well as ethical duty to preserve confidences (NMC, 2008). Information should only be shared where necessary. Holding medical records electronically increases the risks of breaching confidentiality (Roscoe, 2008). The information collected about patients belongs to them and only those who need to know should access this information and be able to justify why they are using this information.

Scenario 12 considers a third party asking for information about a patient.

Patients have the right to see personal information and have it corrected if it is wrong. This could relate to an incorrect diagnosis. For example a young lady recently requested that a diagnosis be removed as it was not proven following a scan (anecdotal). Every practice must have a data controller who is responsible for processing and securing personal data. It is useful to know who has this role in the practice.

Data protection for children under the age of 16 years

The legal guardian of children under 16 years has the right to see their children's records without consent of the child. However, if the child is considered competent and does not wish their parents to know about information in their records, the nurse should take account of this and should not release this information without consent.

Beware of accidentally breaching confidentiality during a joint consultation (Roscoe, 2008). This can occur, for example, when a parent accompanies a child for a travel vaccine, and sees a note about contraception on the computer screen.

There may be a note on the records stating that the patient does not wish their parents to be informed about certain facts. It is essential to position the computer so the only person who can see the screen is the user. However, this is difficult with child and parent present. Ideally the records would be divided into what parent can access, and that which the child wishes to be kept confidential.

If there are any concerns about a particular patient request for information, refer to your employer for advice. Ensure the computer screen does not show the previous patient's records while the next patient enters the room.

Scenario 12

Mrs B has attended for her routine smear. While in the surgery she asked for her 20 year-old daughter's swab results. The nurse explained that she could not disclose this information. Mrs B became aggressive and would not accept the explanation.

There was no record that Mrs B's daughter had given her consent for any information to be divulged to a named person. Mrs B thought that as the nurse knew the family she would be able to share the results.

The nurse was aware of the close family dynamics. The results might have suggested a sexually transmitted infection that the patient wished to remain confidential. Disclosing the information would have been a breach of confidentiality, against the NMC (2008) Code. This could have resulted in a formal complaint against the nurse.

Although it would appear to be harmless to tell Mrs B that the swab results were all negative, this cannot occur without patient consent. The nurse followed good practice by refusing to disclose information. The daughter can give written consent for her mother to receive investigation results. This must then be clearly documented in the patient records.

Caldicott principles

A Caldicott Guardian is a senior person in each NHS organisation who is responsible for safeguarding the confidentiality of patient information (NHS Executive, 1999). The need for safeguarding confidentiality cannot be overstated.

Summary

The nurse must consider all aspects of ethics within the consultation. Consent must be informed, even when it is implied. A few seconds to explain a procedure, or the potential outcome of a procedure, can change a patient's mind. Always act in the patient's best interests, acting as advocate where necessary. The NMC Code should guide each nurse's actions (NMC, 2008).

Key points

- Gain informed consent prior to procedure
- All consultations must be confidential, unless patient safety is compromised
- Complete documentation at the end of each consultation.

Beauchamp T, Childress J (2001) *Principles of Biomedical Ethics* 5th edn. Oxford University Press, New York

Chadwick R, Tadd W (1992) *Ethics and Nursing Practice*. Macmillan, London

Edwards M (2008) *The Informed Practice Nurse* 2nd edn. Wiley, Chichester

Department of Health (1997) *The Caldicott Committee: Report on the Review of Patient-identifiable Information*. HMSO, London

NHS Executive (1999) *Caldicott Guardians. Health Service Circular 1999/012*. The Stationery Office, London

Nursing and Midwifery Council (2007) *Record keeping*. NMC, London

Nursing and Midwifery Council (2008) *The Code. Standards of conduct, performance and ethics for nurses and midwives*. NMC, London

Partners in advocacy (2007) About Advocacy www.partnersinadvocacy.org.uk accessed 21/1/2009

Roscoe T (2008) Computers, confidentiality and the Data Protection Act. BMJ Learning. www.bmj.com/learning/flow.html... accessed 26/1/2009

Smith T (2009) Last word: "While I am here". *United Kingdom Casebook* **17**(1): 26

CHAPTER 4

The patient-centred consultation

The most important person in the consultation is the patient. It is their agenda and not the nurse's that is important. The patient is not interested in targets or whether the nurse has managed to complete all the relevant paper work. He wants to know his health concerns are noted and answered, and also wants the nurse's undivided attention. This chapter explores issues relating to patient-centred care.

Developing the consultation

As discussed in Chapter 2, good communication is vital to enable patients to make informed decisions, supported by access to evidence-based information and education.

A structured approach can improve the consultation. Patients must share their concerns and the nurse must be satisfied that all the vital points have been fully discussed during each time-limited consultation. Brant (2007) noted that although there is an interchange of information between the patient and health professional, the relationship is initiated by the patient and is therefore patient-centred. However, patients who are invited to the surgery, for example, for immunisations, might argue that in these instances the nurse initiates the consultation.

The Calgary-Cambridge framework is used in medical schools and can be applied to nurse consultations. The five main areas of a consultation are:

- Initiation
- Information gathering
- Physical examination
- Explanation and planning
- Session closure.

This framework is loosely followed in the following text. *Box 4.1* incorporates these areas into a patient centred consultation. The nurse must identify:

- Why has the patient presented? Is it a routine hypertension review or a new event such as referral from the optician following an eye examination?
- Does the patient have a particular concern? Is there a hidden agenda? For example, although the patient has presented for his/her hypertension review, he/she is worried about his risk of cardiovascular disease and wishes to discuss his/her family history.

The greatest single problem in consultations is the failure to let the patient tell their story, with most doctors interrupting their patients after 15–18 seconds (Robertson, 2008). Does this reflect the nurse consultation? Developing consultation skills is discussed in Chapter 10.

There needs to be shared understanding between the patient and nurse, for example, explain why drinking too much alcohol can increase blood pressure. Be open if a problem is not within your skills, such as a mental health problem. Refer the patient to the relevant colleague.

It is important to appreciate that the patient is often his own 'expert'. Someone with a chronic disease can usually tell when something is different about their health. This also applies to parents when they say, for example, their child is 'not himself'.

Box 4.1 A patient-centred consultation

- Establish the initial rapport
- Identify the reason for the consultation
- Explore the problem
  - use open questions
  - actively listen
  - search for cues
  - use language the patient understands, and whenever possible use the patient's own words
  - recall and reflect what the patient says
- Establish the patient's perspective
  - concerns
  - expectations
- Build the relationship
  - involve the patient in the management plan for the condition
  - ensure the patient fully understands the action plan
  - arrange a review date

(Source: Brant, 2007; Lloyd and Craig, 2007; Miles, 2008; Robertson, 2008)

Opening the consultation

Having greeted the patient and introduced yourself, it is time to start the consultation. There are many ways of starting a consultation. *'How can I help you'*, or *'What can I do for you'* are questions commonly used by doctors. These are appropriate for patients who consult infrequently, but probably not for those seen regularly. However, be aware that even the regular patient can present with a different concern, and may open the consultation with a spontaneous, unguarded remark, known as a 'curtain-raising' phrase, that provides valuable clues to other concerns (Kaufman, 2008). Nurses often use more informal approaches, such as *'Hello, isn't it cold today? Come in and sit down'*. This, coupled with the smile and eye contact, engages the patient and encourages the patient to start their story. The consultation follows a systematic format (*Box 4.2*).

Box 4.2 Example of a systematic consultation

- Welcome: rapport
- Questions: history, concerns
- Listening: non-verbal cues and body language
- Response: clarify, reflect and summarise
- Explanation: give important information first
- Closure: action plan and review

Taking a patient's history

All practice nurses will undertake some history taking during their daily consultations as part of their general assessment procedure. This may be ascertaining the cause of a leg wound or undertaking a health check. As noted previously, the environment should be accessible, appropriately equipped, free from distractions and safe for the patient and nurse.

Scenario 1 presents a more detailed consultation, in order to gain information and complete a template.

Taking a sexual history

Some nurses are not comfortable taking a patient's sexual history, although this is often an integral part of many consultations related to contraception and related sexual health.

If the patient appears anxious, reiterate that any questions are relevant to the consultation and that absolute confidentiality will be maintained.

Be non-judgemental about the patient's sexual orientation or sexual practices (Suresh and Suresh, 2008). Give the patient the opportunity to talk freely and discuss their concerns, allowing them to write down any points if they are too embarrassed to speak about them. Reassure the patient that they can return at a later date to discuss any issues if they prefer. Pay special attention to any history of sexual abuse (Suresh and Suresh, 2008).

Scenario 1

The new patient check

Welcome
The nurse calls Stephen S in the waiting room, welcomes him, introduces herself and directs him to the consulting room. She confirms his name, date of birth and address to avoid confusion when there is more than one patient with the same name. This is especially relevant when son and father have the same first name.

Purpose of the visit
The nurse ensures Stephen knows the purpose of the new patient check — that is, to have a record of his health history while awaiting his medical records, as these may not be available for several weeks.

Consent
Although it is assumed that Stephen has given his implied consent to the health check as he has attended the appointment, the nurse asks for his consent before undertaking any physical intervention, such as blood pressure reading.

Medical history
A health check would include past and current medical history, and any medications he is taking. Knowledge of relevant family history for at least two generations, including cardiovascular disease (CVD), diabetes and cancer is important to put Stephen's current health concerns into perspective. His father has Type 2 diabetes and hypertension.

Current health
The nurse elicits important information about his lifestyle and immunisation status. Stephen admits to binge drinking at weekends, although he does not smoke and tries to eat a balanced diet and take regular exercise. His blood pressure is normal and his body mass index is less than 25.

Explanation of any untoward findings
The nurse explains the dangers of binge drinking, offers advice and discusses Stephen's risk of CVD with his father's medical history. She uses clear, unambiguous language to ensure Stephen fully understands how alcohol damages the liver and is related to high blood pressure. A shared approach is used to plan how to reduce the binge drinking to a safer level.

Identify concerns
The nurse asks Stephen if he has concerns he wishes to discuss, either with her or the doctor. He volunteers the information that he wishes to be screened for sexually transmitted infections (STIs) as he had unprotected sexual intercourse recently when drunk. He has checked the internet for information and is aware of the range of STIs he might have contracted. He is also worried about his risk of diabetes.

Response and summarising
The nurse reflects on what has been said, summarises the health concerns, and ensures she has not misunderstood or misrepresented any details during the consultation, allowing Stephen the opportunity to clarify any points prior to documentation.

Closure
The nurse offers Stephen a leaflet with details of the local genitourinary medicine (GUM) clinic, and how to self-refer. Signposting is a common skill that enables patients to access the correct service. She also books him an appointment for a fasting blood sugar to exclude diabetes, having explained the procedure and how to access the results. Review will be at Stephen's instigation.

Documentation
All details are contemporaneously documented. This includes all findings, advice given, signposting, booked investigations and review details.

Negotiating a mutual plan of action

Some patients want to be involved in their care plan, others prefer to be non-autonomous and accept what they are advised.

Tips on how to negotiate a mutual plan of action are listed in *Box 4.3*. Scenario 2 exemplifies the simplicity of a negotiated plan of action.

Box 4.3 Tips on how to negotiate a mutual plan of action

1. Discuss the available options, for example, no action, self-care, medication
2. Provide risks and benefits of each option
3. Get the patient's views on the options
4. Accept the patient's views but advocate alternatives if necessary
5. Find out the patient's concerns
6. Take the patient's lifestyle and beliefs into consideration
7. Ask the patient what they want to do
8. Agree on a plan of action
9. Check with the patient that they are satisfied
10. Implement the plan
11. Arrange a follow up appointment

(Source: Prentice, 2008)

Scenario 2

The practice nurse welcomed Amy and invited her to sit down. It transpired that Amy wished to start the oral contraceptive pill. The nurse took a full medical history to exclude contraindications and then asked Amy why she had chosen the pill.

Amy: 'My boyfriend doesn't like using condoms and my friends are on the pill.'

Using the tips in Box 4.3, the nurse continued the consultation. Amy was sexually active, so some form of contraception was essential (1).

The nurse discussed a range of contraceptive methods, with their risks and benefits, and supported the information with leaflets (2).

Amy was not aware of the various options and was pleased to be given a choice (3).

Amy did not really want any hormones, but was scared of becoming pregnant (4 and 5).

Amy was in a stable relationship, but smoked 10 cigarettes a day and had a body mass index of 29. The risk of smoking with the combined pill was emphasised, and the benefits of condom use stressed (6).

Having been given all the information, Amy was unsure what action she wished to take (7).

The agreed action plan was for Amy to take the information home, to re-read and discuss with her boyfriend. She would return on the first day of her next period if she wanted the long acting reversible contraceptive injection or the pill (8).

The nurse checked that Amy understood and was satisfied with the plan (9).

Amy attended the following week on day 1 of her period, requesting the injection. She also asked for a supply of condoms (10).

Amy put a reminder for the next injection into her mobile phone calendar (11).

Changing priorities

Consultations must be flexible to meet patient need. Although they attend for one condition, another might take priority. It is not unreasonable to re-book for the initial condition in these instances. Consider scenario 3.

Scenario 3

Mrs O was an 88-year-old woman who attended for her annual review and spirometry for chronic obstructive pulmonary disease (COPD), escorted by her nephew. The nurse collected Mrs O from the waiting room, and noted her breathlessness and pallor as she walked to the consulting room. It was apparent that Mrs O would not manage the spirometry, so the consultation then focused on the pallor. Was the breathless due to the COPD or another cause? A review of the patient notes and letters highlighted that Mrs O was known to suffer from periodic anaemia. Pulse and blood pressure were within normal limits. Mrs O had no appetite and had lost weight. There was no history of bleeding. Following a joint review with the GP, blood was taken for a range of tests, including full blood count. A review appointment was made with the nurse for the following week.

The laboratory phoned the blood result to the practice that afternoon. Mrs O had a haemoglobin reading of 8g/mml. The doctor visited Mrs O at home to explain the results and arrange hospital admission, which Mrs O refused, preferring to be treated with iron tablets.

> The family and GP acknowledged her autonomy and allowed Mrs O to stay at home and be supported by her family and the medical and nursing team.
>
> The respiratory assessment was deferred until Mrs O was sufficiently well.

In this instance the initial appointment was deferred as the least important health issue on this occasion. The nurse had known Mrs O for several years, and thus was able to recognise her abnormal breathing pattern and pallor. Had the nurse used an automatic call system she may have missed the extra exertion needed by Mrs O to reach the consulting room. Her consultation skills included the ability to continue the rapport, and use both verbal and non-verbal cues to identify that Mrs O was unwell.

Patient autonomy

The professional trend towards negotiated, autonomous nurse-patient health care has enabled a move away from the old paternalistic methods where health professionals knew what was best for the patient, although it is important to recognise that some patients still prefer to follow instructions without information, accepting the nurse's advice. The patient's role is changing from one of grateful recipient to active consumer. It has been argued that although completely autonomous decision-making is a myth, the person seeking informed consent should allow the individual the freedom to make his own choice, although deciding a person's autonomous interests is a difficult matter.

The NMC Code (2008a) stresses the nurses' role in respecting patients' involvement in planning and delivery of care. This is reinforced in the scenario above when Mrs O refused hospital admission against the doctor's recommendation. Nurses have a duty to inform patients of their rights and assist them to ask questions and express their opinions.

The nurse has a duty to respect patients who prefer to be non-autonomous and passive in their care, preferring the nurse or doctor to make all the decisions about their care. Patients should be offered information about their disease, treatment and general management, and allowed to accept or reject this offer.

The physical aspect of the consultation

Nurses are in physical contact with their patients for almost all consultations. Besides the physical tasks such as wound management or cervical smears, they touch the patient while taking a blood pressure, shaking hands and having a hug. There are several areas to consider before and during a consultation where physical contact occurs.

Infection control

During all consultations it is essential to be aware of the recommended infection control measures. Patients can be reassured by seeing the nurse following these basic recommendations. All nurses should be aware of correct hand washing techniques. Alcohol hand rub is an alternative to hand washing in some instances. Kept on the desk, this acts as a reminder to use regularly, especially before and after simple tasks such as checking blood pressures. Patients are often used to the use of hand rub in hospitals, and can be reassured seeing the practice nurse following the same standards. Let the patient see single use equipment disposed of after use to reassure them that all possible steps are taken to reduce cross infection.

Preserving dignity

Many practice nurse consultations do not require a physical examination. However, within the varied remit of the practice nurse role, patients are often examined in different scenarios; for example, a lady may need to remove her tights to enable the nurse to examine and dress a leg ulcer. Women are subjected to intimate examinations when they attend for cervical screening and vaginal examinations, although nurses will less commonly examine male genitalia. It is impossible to diagnose a skin rash unless the skin is exposed. The patient might proffer an arm or lower leg to demonstrate a rash, whereas the trunk and whole limbs should be examined. Vaginal discharge exemplifies the need for a physical examination. Examination and swabs for microbiology investigation are necessary for differential diagnosis (Edwards, 2007).

It is essential that the patient consent to any physical examination. This can only occur if the procedure has been explained (see Chapter 3). Allow the patient as much dignity as possible, and ensure privacy if clothing is removed. Close window curtains or blinds, as well as screens or curtains around the bed. This will help reduce patient embarrassment. Explain to the patient that the door is locked for their privacy, and not because you are locking them in! This is particularly relevant when undertaking intimate examinations — it is not uncommon for patients to wander into the wrong consulting room when they are lost.

Allow the patient to remove the minimum amount of clothing if having a smear, while encouraging the patient to expose greater body area when assessing skin conditions. Looking solely at a face cannot assess the extent of acne. The shoulders, chest and back should also be examined. Teenagers may be uncomfortable with this, hence the need for a full explanation and rationale for the examination. Consider the patient's dignity at all times.

The following scenario describes the physical aspect when a woman attends for a cervical smear.

Scenario 4

Miss E has attended for her first smear. The nurse has completed the documentation, explained the rationale behind smears and how Miss E will receive the results. Miss E consented to the procedure and declined a chaperone.

Nurse: 'I need you to remove your tights and pants.' [Locks the door and directs patient to couch, behind curtains.]

Nurse [indicating sheet of bedroll]: 'This is your modesty blanket. Pop it across your tummy when you're ready.' [Indicates the genital region on herself. Allows patient to remove clothing in privacy while assembling equipment.]

Nurse: 'Are you comfortable?' [Adjusts pillow at head of bed. Asks patient to raise knees, ankles together and open legs.]

Nurse: 'I'm just looking at the outside to make sure everything looks normal. It looks fine. I'm now going to put the spec inside you. Is that ok?' [Nurse checks patient's face for non-verbal cues. Patient nods OK.]

Nurse: 'Now I'm going to open the spec and it might feel a little uncomfortable.'

Nurse: 'I'm going to take the smear now, so you'll feel some pressure'. [Takes smear.]

Nurse: 'I'm taking the spec out now.'

[Nurse reassures patient that the cervix appeared satisfactory and reiterated how she would receive the results.]

Nurse: 'Have you any questions?'

Miss E: 'No. Thanks. You've been very kind and explained everything. I was very nervous, but feel fine now.'

This scenario demonstrates good verbal and non-verbal communication skills. The nurse talked her way through the procedure so the patient knew exactly what would happen next. She considered the patient's comfort and dignity. This example can be transferred to almost all physical aspects of a consultation. For example, with ear irrigation as in the scenario below.

Scenario 5

Nurse: 'What can I do for you today?' [Ascertains reason for consultation.]

Patient: 'My ears need syringing.'

Nurse: 'Is it OK if I have a look in your ears?' [Gains patient consent.]

Patient: 'Yes, nurse'

Nurse looks in both ears with otoscope.

Nurse: 'There is wax in the right ear, but the left eardrum is clear. I only need to irrigate the right ear. Have you had them irrigated before?'

Patient: 'Not for a long time.'

Nurse clarifies that the patient has no contraindications to the irrigation, prepares equipment and electric irrigation machine.

Nurse: 'This machine makes a bit of a noise. It sounds like this.' [Lets machine run for a few seconds.]

Nurse: 'Let me know if you have any pain or discomfort or if the water temperature is uncomfortable and I'll stop at once.' [Starts machine.]

Nurse: 'Is that OK?' [Considers patient comfort.]

Patient nods.

Nurse continues with irrigation, removes wax and dries the outer ear.

Nurse: 'I'm just going to check the ears again.' [Looks in ear.]

> Nurse: 'The drums are clear now. All the wax is out. Your hearing might be muffled for a while until the water has evaporated.' [Explanation of outcome.]
>
> The nurse then ensured the patient had no side effects from the ear irrigation, completed the documentation and closed the consultation.
>
> The nurse gained consent for procedure, ensured there were no contraindications to proceed and managed to remove the wax without the need for a further appointment. She ensured the patient was informed at all stages of the procedure.

The need for good communication skills during a physical examination or procedure cannot be overstated.

Chaperones

A chaperone is a guide or companion who is present to ensure propriety or restrict activity. Nurses should consider being accompanied by a chaperone when undertaking an intimate examination or procedure. This is to reassure the patient, avoid misunderstanding and, in rare cases, protect against allegations of improper behaviour. An experienced chaperone will identify unusual or unacceptable behaviour on the part of the nurse.

The Nursing and Midwifery Council states that people have the right to request a chaperone when undergoing any procedure or examination. If a chaperone cannot be provided, the person must be informed and asked whether they wish to continue with the procedure or examination. Their decision should be noted in their records (NMC, 2008b).

The Royal College of Nursing (RCN) offers guidance about the role of chaperones (RCN, 2008).

Principles of good practice in chaperoning
When considering the appropriateness of a chaperone, the nurse should adhere to the following principles of good practice:

* All patients, regardless of age, gender, ethnic background, culture, sexual orientation, or mental status have the right to have their privacy and dignity respected.
* Patients should be offered a chaperone or be invited to have a relative or friend with them during any consultation, examination or procedure. Their personal preference should be documented in their clinical record.
* In order that patients may exercise their right to request the presence

of a chaperone, a full explanation of the consultation, examination or procedure to be carried out should be given to the patient, followed by a check to ensure that the patient has received and understood a sufficient degree of information.

- Record that permission has been obtained in the patient notes.
- If the patient prefers to undergo a consultation, examination or procedure without the presence of a chaperone, their decision should be respected and documented in the clinical record.
- The patient should be informed if a chaperone is unavailable (either due to unforeseen circumstances or an emergency situation) and they should be asked whether or not they consent to the consultation, examination or procedure going ahead without a chaperone. If they prefer, they should be offered the option of postponing the consultation, examination or procedure until one is available.
- Patients should be encouraged to maintain independence and self-care as far as is practicable, for example, by undressing themselves.
- The NHS Clinical Governance Support Team advises it is good practice to offer all patients a chaperone for any consultation, examination or procedure where the patient feels one is required.

A nurse or another member of the healthcare team who acts as a chaperone can act as advocate for the patient, helping to explain what will happen during the examination or procedure and the reasons why. They can reassure the patient and safeguard against any unnecessary discomfort, pain, humiliation or intimidation. In each situation a culture of openness between patients and health care professional should be actively encouraged (RCN, 2008).

The General Medical Council (GMC) also offers guidance for doctors. This guidance is also relevant for nurses when undertaking intimate examinations (GMC, 2001). The GMC advise that a clinician should:

- Explain to the patient why an examination is necessary and give the patient an opportunity to ask questions.
- Explain what the examination will involve, in a way the patient can understand, so that the patient has a clear idea of what to expect, including any potential pain or discomfort.
- Obtain the patient's permission before the examination and be prepared to discontinue the examination if the patient asks you to. You should record that permission has been obtained.
- Keep discussion relevant and avoid unnecessary personal comments.
- Give the patient privacy to undress and dress, and use drapes to maintain the patient's dignity. Do not assist the patient in removing clothing unless you have clarified with them that your assistance is required.

It has been reported that the new emphasis on chaperones creates pressure on already hard-pressed resources as a person who is asked to chaperone is taken away from his or her own work.

Stott (2008) reported that male patients appear to decline the offer of a chaperone more than women, and noted that in some practices if a female refuses a chaperone for an examination by a male clinician, the examination must be deferred until a female practitioner can do it. This may be less common in general practice where most nurses are female. It has also been reported that 72% of female medical students and 29% of male students experienced at least one instance of patient initiated sexual behaviour (Stott, 2008). Practice nurses probably do not report these instances, but there is a case for completing significant event reports when this occurs.

Scenarios 6 and 7 are examples of the importance of using a chaperone in practice for the protection of the nurse.

Scenario 6

Miss P attended for a routine smear. The nurse took a full history and was ready to undertake the smear. She asked Miss P to remove her underwear behind the curtains then lie on the couch. When the nurse entered the area Miss P was completely naked on the couch.

Miss P: 'You can do what you like with me.'

Why did it happen?
Although the nurse made it clear that Miss P was only to remove her underwear, she did not provide a modesty drape to cover her genitalia. The nurse was totally unprepared for this reaction.

What action was taken?
The nurse left the area and asked a colleague to act as chaperone. She also suggested that Miss P partially redressed.

What could have happened?
Miss P could have made an allegation of improper behaviour against the nurse.

Reflection
The nurse was not to know that Miss P would undress completely, which was wholly inappropriate for the procedure. In hindsight she could have sensitively supervised Miss P undressing and handed her the modesty drape before she had time to undress fully. She made sure she was not alone with Miss P during the procedure.

Scenario 7

Sam was a 17-year-old boy who attended for a course of vaccinations. At the last appointment he mentioned he was worried about a spot on his testicle.

The nurse asked Sam if he would like to see a doctor, but he was happy for her to examine him. The nurse agreed to check the area. Sam lay on the couch and exposed his genitals. The nurse had the necessary skills and knowledge, and was comfortable undertaking the examination. The nurse reassured Sam that the spot was a harmless fatty lump.

What could have happened?
Sam could have made a complaint against the nurse for improper behaviour. As there was no witness, it would have been his word against hers. The worst scenario would be suspension and disciplinary investigation.

Reflection
In future the nurse decided to always ask for a chaperone when examining a male patient.

Who can be a chaperone?

A practice staff member may not seem neutral to the patient, while a family member might not be suitable from the practitioner's point of view (Stott, 2008). The GMC (2001) state that the chaperone should be familiar with the examination being performed and should be able to comfort the patient, respect their dignity and preserve confidentiality. The chaperone would usually be of the same sex as the patient to protect the patient from vulnerability and embarrassment.

In an intimate examination the chaperone should stand at the head of the bed, with the examination area covered by a modesty drape. Men who accompany their partners, for example if the woman is disabled, or when an interpreter is needed, usually sit outside the curtains, maintaining the women's privacy. In this instance, ask yourself if this is really an adequate chaperone as the patient standing or sitting outside the curtains would not be able to witness the examination.

All staff should have an understanding of the role of the chaperone and the procedures for raising concerns.

Patient preferences

In a study by Khann and Kirkman (2000) a clear majority (107 *vs* 19) of community clinic users preferred to be alone with the woman doctor or nurse during an internal examination. There was no significant difference in preference or strength of feeling when analysed by age, ethnicity or previous experience.

Osmond et al (2007) undertook a study into chaperones in sexual health medicine. Acceptance of a chaperone was highest among Asian patients, but most patients did not want a chaperone. They concluded that those who do would prefer for a chaperone to be offered, rather than for it to be routine, supporting the recommendation that all patients should be offered a chaperone for intimate examinations.

Issues specific to religion/ethnicity or culture

It is important to maintain dignity and to limit the amount of undressing for an examination as noted above. It would be unwise to proceed with any examination if the nurse is unsure that the patient understands what is going to happen due to a language barrier. If an interpreter is available, they may be able to double as an informal chaperone. This is discussed more fully in Chapter 9.

Children

If a minor presents in the absence of a parent or guardian, the nurse must ascertain if they are capable of understanding the need for examination. In these cases it would be advisable for consent to be secured and a formal chaperone to be present for any intimate examinations (Department of Health, 1999).

Registrant/client abuse

An important but often neglected issue which can occur during a consultation relates to registrant/client relationships and the prevention of abuse (NMC, 2008c). The reader is recommended to download this guidance or request a hard copy from the Nursing and Midwifery Council. The document relates to physical, psychological and verbal abuse (see *Box 4.4*). Consider how all these examples can unconsciously slip into a consultation.

Box 4.4 Examples of registrant/client abuse

Psychological abuse
Mocking
Ignoring
Coercing
Denying privacy

Verbal abuse
Demeaning
Humiliating
Racist
Sexist
Homophobic
Ageist

Sexual abuse
Touching a client inappropriately
Engaging in sexual discussions that have no relevance to the client's care

Source: NMC (2008c)

Patient expectations

What does the patient expect from a consultation? Should he be told what he wants to hear? These are some of the issues that create personality problems. In these instances it is best to accept that nurses and patients will have differences of opinion, and allow these patients to be reviewed by their preferred health professional.

Some of the issues that can create dissatisfaction during a consultation:
- Disagreeing about goals
- Being forced to accept a plan against their will
- Being made to feel worthless
- Feeling ignored
- Lacking confidence
- Feeling rushed

The above points can be remedied with thought and patient-centred care.

- Goals should be negotiated between the patient and nurse. They should be realistic and achievable.
- Forcing a management plan on a patient against their will is unlikely to lead to adherence and might lead to a breakdown in the nurse-patient relationship.

- The patient should be made to feel the most important person in the consultation. Their views are important and should be considered even if they appear bizarre to the nurse.
- Never ignore what the patient says. Their concerns should be addressed sensitively.
- The nurse who is knowledgeable and uses evidence-based information will infuse confidence into the patient.
- Patients feel they have not been listened to if the consultation is rushed
- Patients like to be talked 'with' and not 'to'.

It has been reported that despite efforts to individualise care and find ways to communicate with patients, many people still report dissatisfying clinical encounters (Hornsten et al, 2005).

Summary

The patient is the key person in the consultation. Consider his needs at all times, and identify his anticipated outcome from the consultation. Have his needs been met? Has he been informed throughout? The nurse must also consider her own position and ensure she is not compromised during a physical examination. Nurses must accept that they can hopefully please most patients some of the time, but cannot please all patients all of the time.

Key points

- The patient is the key person in the consultation.
- Good communication skills are essential
- Chaperones play a key role in risk management

Brant C (2007) The nurse will see you. *Nursing Standard* **22**(13): 62–3

Department of Health (1999) *Working Together to Safeguard Children*. DH, London

Edwards M (2007) Identifying vaginal candiasis. *Practice Nurse* **34**(6): 31–5

Edwards M (2008) *The Informed Practice Nurse* 2nd edn. Wiley, Chichester

General Medical Council (2001) *Chaperones in primary care*. www.gpnotebook.co.uk accesses 23/1/2009

Hornsten A, Lundman B, Selstan E, Sandstrom H (2005) Patient satisfaction with diabetes care. *Journal of Advanced Nursing* **51**(6): 609–17

Kaufman G (2008) Patient assessment: effective consultation and history taking. *Nursing Standard* **23**(4): 50–6

Khann NS, Kirkman R (2000) Intimate examinations: use of chaperones in community-based family planning clinics. *British Journal of Obstetrics and Gynaecology* **107**(1): 130–2

Lloyd H, Craig S (2007) A guide to taking a patient's history. *Nursing Standard* **22**(13): 42–8

Miles J (2008) Effective communication. *Practice Nurse* **35**(2): 42–7

Nursing and Midwifery Council (2008a) *The Code. Standards of conduct, performance and ethics for nurses and midwives*. NMC, London

Nursing and Midwifery Council (2008b) *Chaperoning*. NMC, London

Nursing and Midwifery Council (2008c) *Registrant/client relationships and the prevention of abuse*. NMC, London

Osmond MK, Copas AJ, Newey C et al (2007) The use of chaperones for intimate examinations: the patient perspective based on an anonymous questionnaire. *International Journal of STD & AIDS* **18**(10): 667–71

Prentice P (2008) How practice nurse and patients can help each other. *BMJ Learning. Practice Nurse CPD*. http://learning.bmj.com accessed 21/1/2008

Robertson K (2008) The importance of communication skills. *Practice nurse CPD. BMJ Learning*. http://learning.bmj.com accessed 20/10/08

Royal College of Nursing (2008) *Chaperoning: The role of the nurse and the rights of patients*. London, RCN

Stott D (2008) Chaperones for intimate examinations. *Student.BMJ*. http://student bmj.com/ phprint.php accessed 22/2/12009

Suresh K, Suresh P (2008) Tips on one to one interactions. *BMJ Learning*. www.learning. bmj.com accessed 21/10.2008

CHAPTER 5

Children and adolescents

Practice nurses will encounter children and adolescents throughout their working week. The nurse must be conversant with the legal aspects of consent and confidentiality as an integral part of her consultation skills. The Children's Act 2004 advised that childrens' wishes and feelings regarding their care need to be acknowledged. This chapter will examine some of the ethical and legal issues relating to this patient group and offer tips for consulting with children and young people.

Confidentiality

Young people under 16 years old have as great a right to confidentiality as any other patient. Even if the person is not judged mature enough to consent to treatment, the consultation itself can still remain confidential.

Consent to treatment in children

In English law the nurse must obtain informed consent before she can examine or treat a patient. This requires that:

- The nurse gives relevant information about the intervention
- The patient is competent to make the decision
- The patient decides voluntarily.

Involving children

The key issue in child consent is that a child who is capable of making a reasoned decision has a right to be involved in the decision-making process. Children need to be fully informed in the same way as any other patient. If they are old enough to explain their feelings, it is worth asking the child why they have come and ask them to describe the problem (Gregory and Richards, 2006).

In a study by Martenson and Fagerskiold (2008) children showed trust and expressed a wish to use self-determination. They reported that age-appropriate information and participation were prerequisites for allowing children the opportunity to make competent decisions about their own care.

Competence

The nurse must establish whether the child is legally competent, that is, has the competence to give consent. If the child is not deemed legally competent, consent must be obtained from someone with parental responsibility.

Children under the age of 16
The Fraser Guidelines (previously Gillick competence) states that children under 16 years can give valid consent to treatment if they have sufficient maturity and intelligence to understand the nature and implications of the proposed treatment. The Children Act 1989, Section 3(5) provides guidance for nurses dealing with emergencies in primary care when a minor is accompanied by someone without parental responsibility, for example a school teacher or a carer. Safeguarding or promoting the child's welfare is paramount. Requests for confidentiality must be respected, although the nurse should encourage the young person to involve their parents in their care.

The Fraser Guidelines provide criteria for health professionals to establish whether a girl under 16 years is competent to consent to contraceptive treatment. The nurse must be satisfied that:

- The young person will understand the nurse's advice
- The young person cannot be persuaded to inform their parents
- The young person is likely to begin, or to continue having, sexual intercourse with or without contraceptive treatment
- Unless the young person receives contraceptive treatment their physical or mental health, or both, are likely to suffer
- The young person's best interests require them to receive contraceptive advice or treatment with or without parental consent.

This guidance can be applied to other scenarios, including vaccinations. Parents might refuse to have a child vaccinated as a baby, but the young person can then seek treatment when of an age to give informed consent without parental consent.

Scenarios 1 and 2 relates to the non-consenting child.

Scenario 1

Jed attended as a walk-in emergency at lunchtime. He was 15 years old and unaccompanied. The nurse welcomed him and ushered him into the consulting room. Jed's right hand was bandaged with a dirty handkerchief. The nurse removed the dressing, at the same time gaining the history. The wound was a 3-day old burn which had a broken blister. The wound needed to be cleaned and dressed, and a tetanus vaccine was recommended.

Why did it happen?
Jed was a non-attendee at school and was often left to his own devices. He appeared to be an independent boy. He had not been vaccinated as a baby.

What action was taken?
The nurse assessed Jed and established that he was competent to give consent to the treatment, and also to start a primary course of vaccinations. She explained why these were recommended and discussed the minor side-effects that he might experience. She then dressed the wound and administered the first diphtheria, tetanus and polio vaccination. Follow-up appointments were made for dressings and further vaccinations. These were written on a card as reminders. Jed was encouraged to share this information with his parents.

Implications for practice
Jed might not have returned for treatment if asked to attend with a parent. The wound required immediate dressing to prevent infection. The vaccinations would protect Jed from some infections and also contribute to herd immunity. The nurse had assessed Jed and gained his informed consent to the treatment. The care was in his best interests.

Reflection
The nurse would have preferred a parent to have accompanied Jed, but as he always attended follow-up appointments unaccompanied, she realised that she had made the right decision. Jed received regular care, the wound healed and he completed the course of injections, and also agreed to the measles, mumps and rubella vaccine.

Scenario 2

Ben was booked in to see the nurse for his school leaving booster injection at age 14 years. He attended with his mother. The nurse greeted him and invited him to sit down. Ben remained standing with his arms crossed across his chest. The nurse explained what the injection was, and the protection it conferred. She explained that there was minimal pain, but the arm would probably ache for a few hours. Ben refused to remove his jumper. His mother became angry and threatening, which made the nurse uncomfortable and Ben more uncooperative.

Why did it happen?
Ben knew why he was at the surgery, but changed his mind. He did not consent to the injection.

What action was taken?
The nurse explained to Ben and his mother that she would not give the injection without Ben's consent. She suggested that Ben went away and thought about the injection, and return during the school holidays if he changed his mind.

Implications for practice
If his mother had restrained Ben and the nurse administered the injection without Ben's consent, this could have been construed as assault. Ben had the mental capacity to understand the procedure. If the nurse tried to give the injection and Ben struggled, the needle might have broken and embedded under the skin. This was not a risk the nurse was prepared to take. In addition, the nurse might be hurt in the struggle.

Reflection
Although Ben's mother had given her consent, it was apparent that Ben was not prepared for the injection. If a child fully understands the implications of the vaccine and has a valid reason for refusing, the nurse should heed the child's request. Ben was given the opportunity to return when he was psychologically prepared. The nurse considered both Ben's and her own personal safety.

Children aged 16 and 17

Once children reach the age of 16 they are presumed by law to be competent to give consent for medical treatment (Department of Health, 2001). It is good practice to encourage young people to involve their parents/carers in decisions about their care, but confidentiality must always be respected. However, in cases where the child is at risk, for example from abuse, the nurse must disclose this information with the relevant authorities (NMC, 2008).

Children are dependent on their parents or carers for their health and safety. Most parents look to health professionals to help them make the right choices to ensure that their children grow up with healthy lives. The Best Interest Standard refers to the legal assumption that parents act in their children's best interests (Beauchamp and Childress, 2001). To be able to consent, a parent must have sufficient information to weigh up risks and benefits of a procedure. Failure to provide this information may lead to the consent being invalid.

It is not uncommon for a minor to refuse treatment, for example an immunisation, but for the parent to give consent. Legally, if the parents have given consent the nurse may give the injection, although forcing the child to be immunised against his will can be construed as criminal assault. If the child fully understands the implications of the vaccine and has a valid reason for refusing, the nurse should heed the child's request. See scenario 3.

Scenario 3

Amanda, aged 17 years, attended the asthma clinic for her annual review accompanied by her mother. The nurse noticed that she had only had one measles, mumps and rubella (MMR) vaccine. She explained that the recommendations are for two injections, discussed the rationale for this and that she appeared to have missed the second injection. The nurse also explained the dangers of a woman contracting rubella in pregnancy and offered to give the injection during the consultation. Amanda's mother encouraged her to have it, but Amanda said she was not prepared for it and refused. The nurse respected Amanda's decision, but gave her a leaflet about the MMR and suggested she came during the next school holidays.

Parental responsibility

In England and Wales, the parents of a child who are married to each other at the time of the birth, or if they have jointly adopted a child, both have parental responsibility. Parents do not lose parental responsibility if they divorce, and this applies to both the resident and the non-resident parent.

However this is not automatically the case for unmarried parents. According to current law, a mother always has parental responsibility for her child (Directgov, 2009). A father, however, has this responsibility only if he is married to the mother when the child is born or has acquired legal responsibility for his child through one of these three routes:

- After 1 December 2003, by jointly registering the birth of the child with the mother
- By a parental responsibility agreement with the mother
- By a parental responsibility order, made by a court.

Living with the mother, even for a long time, does not give a father parental responsibility, and if the parents are not married parental responsibility does not always pass to the natural father if the mother dies. If consent from someone with parental responsibility is required, only one individual needs to be approached. The Children's Act 1989 outlines who else has parental responsibility:

- The child's legally appointed guardian, appointed either by a court or by a parent with parental responsibility in the event of their own death
- A person in whose favour a court has made a residency order concerning the child
- A local authority designated in a care order in respect of the child
- A local authority or other authorised person who holds an emergency protection order in respect of the child.

Foster parents, grandparents and parents under the age of 16 do not automatically have parental responsibility. If the parent is under the age of 16, they must have proven Fraser competence before they can give consent on behalf of their child.

Children who are wards of court require their 'important steps' to be approved by the court. It is helpful to keep a scanned copy of the ward papers in the medical records to guide the nurse on what treatment can be offered without reference to the court.

The Children Act 1989 Section 3(5) provides guidance for nurses dealing with emergencies in primary care when a minor is accompanied by someone without parental responsibility, for example a school teacher or a carer. Safeguarding or promoting the child's welfare is paramount.

Devolving parental responsibility

Parents can devolve responsibility to consent to others, for example grandparents or childminders, for interventions such as emergency care or treatment of minor illnesses. This consent does not need to be in writing, and the nurse does not have to consult the parents unless there is a cause to believe parent's views would differ significantly (Department of Health, 2001). This is particularly relevant when undertaking child immunisation, when a foster parent, childminder or relative brings the baby or child. Bringing the child for immunisation is seen as implied consent, but it is important to ensure that consent is informed. Written consent is not a legal requirement of the Children Act 1989 but is helpful for nurses in cases of litigation. The importance of gaining informed consent is demonstrated in the following scenario.

Scenario 4

Baby Jane is booked into baby clinic for her 13-month measles, mumps and rubella (MMR) and pneumococcal booster. She is brought by her paternal grandmother but has no letter with written consent from a parent. It is practice procedure to have signed consent from a parent before immunisation. The nurse asks whether Jane's parents had any questions about the MMR, but grandma does not know. Informed consent cannot be assumed in this instance. The nurse asks grandma to telephone Jane's mother to gain verbal consent, which is given. This is documented on the patient records, grandma signs the immunisation sheet and the vaccinations are given.

Although nurses can administer immunisation without documented consent, they need to be aware of potential problems. In the above scenario, Baby Jane's father might have agreed to the MMR, but the mother may not. However, consent from only one person with parental responsibility is legally required.

Consultation skills when a parent attends with a young child

Environment

A welcoming environment is essential when consulting with children. Children quickly become bored so it helps to have a selection of toys in the room to distract them while talking to the parent of a young child. When addressing the child, sit at the same level as them to gain eye contact. Spend a few moments at the beginning of the consultation building a rapport with the child. Asking the name of a teddy bear or about the picture on their shirt or dress can help put the child at ease. Try to use terms the child will understand, for example 'wee wee' and 'poo', and do not tell white lies. Parents should also be honest with their children. The following scenario puts this into context.

Scenario 5

Harry enters the room with his mother. The nurse is aware that Harry is due his pre-school booster injection. Harry stands close to his mother.

Nurse: 'Hello Harry. Who's that on your T-shirt?' [Starts to make Harry feel at ease]

Harry: 'Bob the Builder'

Nurse: 'Tell me what he does'

Ben chatters away. Nurse clarifies reason for visit, ascertains that Harry is well, explains the side effects of the injections and gains written consent for the vaccinations.

Nurse [to mother]: 'Does Harry know why he is here?'

Mother: 'No. I thought you could tell him.'

Nurse: 'You can tell him while I prepare the injections.' [Passes responsibility to mother.]

Mother [to Harry]: 'The nurse is just going to give you a needle in your arm. It won't hurt.'

Nurse: 'It will hurt just a little. But not as much as when you fall over.' [Don't tell a lie.]

Harry is prepared and sits on his mother's lap holding Pooh Bear, who usually sits on a shelf. The nurse fetches a colleague and administers the two injections

---

simultaneously. This reduces the likelihood of Harry resisting the second injection. Harry's mother gives consent for the nurse to offer him a sugar-free lolly as a reward after the event. The consultation ends.

How would Harry have felt if he had believed that the injection would not hurt, and then it did? He would lose trust in both his mother and the nurses who administered the injections. All injections hurt to some extent, so be honest and say so.

Communication with children

It is important to gain an accurate understanding of the child's perspective of their condition. They are experts on themselves and only they can offer certain information. Assessing a child's knowledge level is also important. This could relate to which inhalers they use and why. It may also help the nurse understand why a child does not adhere to a skin care regime.

When the patient is the child it is vital to remember to communicate to the child directly, even though the parent is also a key person. Address the child first, and where possible let the child tell his/her own story. Try to prevent the parent interrupting the story. This is particularly important when asked to see a child who has had a head injury, as shown in scenario 6.

Scenario 6

Nurse: 'Hello, Sam. How old are you now?'

Sam: 'I'm six.'

Nurse: 'Gosh, you are getting old. What happened to you?'

Mother: 'He fell in the playground.'

Nurse: 'I'd like Sam to tell me in his own words please. Sam, can you tell me exactly what happened?'

Sam: 'I was playing football with my friends, and tripped over Joe, and fell.'

Nurse: 'Where do you hurt?'

Sam indicates the back of his head, where a lump has started to develop. The nurse excluded any adverse neurological signs, reassured the mother, advised a cold compress and paracetamol, and gave the mother written head injury instructions.

Nurse: 'If you are at all concerned go straight to accident and emergency.'

Sam was able to recall what had happened at school, so had not lost consciousness, but the nurse could not have ascertained this from mother's intervention. Explain the rationale of questioning the child to the parent, and involve them in the consultation.

Children watch the interaction between the nurse and parent, and will respond positively to the mutual respect shown between the two. Some children are scared and will not allow a nurse near them, either because of a previous painful encounter, or a fear of the unknown. Patience is essential. Smile at the child and talk to them.

Scenario 7

Milly is booked in for a dressing. She is 4 years old.

Nurse: 'Hello, Milly. Hello Mrs Jones. Please sit down.'

Mrs Jones is seated, and Milly stands close, facing her mother.

Nurse: 'I see Milly is booked for a dressing. What happened?'

Mrs Jones: 'Milly tipped over a mug of hot tea and scalded her arm. We went to casualty yesterday and were told to see a nurse today.'

Nurse [to Milly]: 'Can I have a look at your arm please?'

Milly gets closer to mum.

Nurse [to Milly]: ' Can you show me on teddy where the poorly is on your arm?" [Gives Milly a teddy. Milly points to teddy's left arm.]

Nurse: 'Should we show teddy your poorly arm?'

Milly reluctantly proffers her arm which is bandaged from wrist to elbow. Teddy has a look.

Nurse: 'I'm just going to take this off. I'll try not to hurt you.' [Points to bandage.]

Milly looks concerned. The nurse gently removes the bandage and dressing, watching for non-verbal signs of pain.

Nurse [to Milly]: 'You're being very brave.'

Nurse [to Mrs Jones]: 'There's no sign of infection, which is good. I'm going to put some more cream on and I'd like to see Milly again in two days.'

Nurse [to Milly]: 'This cream will be a bit cold.' [Applies cream and dressing.]

Nurse [to Milly]: 'Should I bandage teddy too?'

Milly nods. Nurse bandages teddy.

Nurse completes the bandaging, records the consultation and makes the next mutually convenient appointment.

In this case the nurse directed most of her attention to Milly. She was patient and did not rush the consultation. She used simple language and reassured and praised Milly, whilst giving relevant information to Mrs Jones. Milly's facial expression during the dressing could indicate that the nurse was hurting her. The follow up appointment was made to suit Mrs Jones and the nurse, which is important for continuity of care and allows the nurse to build on her rapport with Milly. Inevitably not all follow up appointments can be with the same nurse in larger practices but where possible this is the ideal situation.

Use lots of eye contact, smiles, fun and laughter where appropriate. Children need to see that the nurse is interested in them and that they care.

Risks associated with disruptive children

Patients should be given realistic expectations of what to expect from a consultation. There are many occasions when children disrupt a consultation. These include accompanying siblings or parents or being present when the parent requires an examination. Nurses should not feel uncomfortable explaining to a patient in layman's terms that the child is compromising the accuracy and safety of the consultation, and asking them to re-book the appointment if necessary. Fortunately it appears to be a minority of children who fit this category but even these few are a danger. If children are disruptive it is reasonable to suggest that the parent re-book to see the nurse.

The following scenario relates to travel vaccinations for a child.

Scenario 8

During a long and difficult consultation for travel injections, when 10-year-old child A refused to have her typhoid vaccination, Mrs L then asked for child A's prescription for malaria prophylaxis. It was difficult to discuss the rationale behind the drug dosage with Mrs L while child A was being disruptive.

It later transpired that an error was made despite the prescription having been checked by three people, including the prescribing doctor and the dispensing pharmacist. This was rectified and the correct drug and dosage delivered to Mrs L.

Mrs L checked the dosage on her home computer, thought the staff had made an error and subsequently reduced the dose of treatment, using 62.5mg as the main dose, instead of the correct 50mg base of chloroquine.

Why did this happen?
Child A was uncooperative and refused the injection. Mrs L eventually persuaded her and the injection was given. However, the delay in administering the injection had resulted in a backlog of patients waiting to see Nurse N. The prescription was prepared under pressure.

What action was taken?
Mrs L later contacted the surgery to say the dose of chloroquine was incorrect and she was giving the child a reduced dose. Nurse N could not contact Mrs L by phone to clarify the dose, but left a message for her to contact the surgery. This was documented in child A's notes. She knew the family well, and was aware that Mrs L would be unlikely to heed any advice, particularly as the holiday was imminent, so did not pursue the matter. Nurse B and the pharmacist completed significant event forms and a practice review was undertaken to prevent reoccurrence of similar incidents.

What could have happened?
Child A was given a sub optimal dose of malaria prophylaxis, thus making her at risk of contracting the disease. Mr and Mrs L are articulate parents who use the internet to supplement other information. However in this instance they put child A's health in jeopardy by not asking the health professionals to clarify any misinformation.

Nurses are often pressurised by demanding patients or when appointments overrun. Children are another issue. Some parents warn their children that they are coming for an injection and it will hurt a little. Others say nothing and expect the nurse to inject without preparation. This creates an atmosphere of fear for the child and stress for the nurse. No nurse is comfortable injecting an unprepared child, and he or she should not be expected to carry out such a procedure in these circumstances. Parents have a responsibility to tell their children what to expect. Ultimately the nurse could refuse to continue the consultation and ask the parent to return another day, explaining that she has other patients waiting to see her as mistakes can be made when people are put under pressure.

In an ideal world all children would be quiet and cooperative. However, the reality is that some children will hide under chairs, run around the room, make a noise and challenge the sanity of staff. If children are uncooperative it is reasonable to suggest that the parent re-book the appointment to see the nurse another time and prepare the child for the procedure. It is unsafe to continue a discussion when the parent is more concerned with the child than listening to the nurse.

In the case above Mrs L did not heed the nurse's information and advice on dosage and frequency of the drug, became confused and accessed another source which she did not fully understand. A team de-brief about this significant event raised several important issues. In hindsight this consultation should have been terminated before the vaccination was given. Mrs L should have taken child A home, re-booked for a later date and thoroughly prepared the child for the injection. As Nurse N had several patients waiting, she should have advised Mrs L that the prescription would be prepared for collection the following day. This would allow Nurse N and the doctor to calculate the dose without duress.

Adolescents

Adolescents can present to the nurse with a variety of conditions (see *Box 5.1*). Adolescents show considerable variation in psychological and physical development so must be treated as individuals. They like to be treated as adults and given due attention to their independence and individuality. Do not patronise older children and adolescents, and let them be involved in both the information gathering and management planning.

Try to engage them in the consultation through a topic of their interest. This is easy when the young man has his skateboard with him, or the youngster wears a T-shirt promoting a certain rock band. The following introduction can make the young person feel more at ease: *'Hello, come in. Please sit down. I see you're into skateboarding. Where do you skate?'*, and then move onto the purpose of the visit.

Most healthcare professionals have little, if any, specific training in how to approach adolescents, with mutual wariness and poor communication common. Robinson (2008) reported that half of adolescents experience problems with the consultation on the infrequent occasions when they do attend. Problems during the consultations include:

- Embarrassment
- Delay in getting an appointment promptly
- Unsympathetic doctor
- Fear of lack of confidentiality.

Although many adolescents attend with a parent they should be offered the opportunity to see the nurse on their own. For example, it can be assumed that a 16-year-old girl who attends for her contraceptive injection accompanied by her mother has an open relationship with her mother. In this instance it might be appropriate to talk about the risk of sexually transmitted infections if there has been a change of partner, however, this would be inappropriate if the girl has had several partners that the mother is unaware of.

It is important to stress that all consultations are confidential, and that the patient's consent must be obtained before information is shared, with some exceptions (NMC, 2008). In the sexual health agenda one of

---

Box 5.1. Common reasons for adolescents consulting a nurse

- Chronic disease such as asthma
- Sexual health, including contraception
- Acne
- Travel advice
- Traumatic sports injuries
- Post operative management

---

the main deterrents regarding seeking help and advice is a fear of lack of confidentiality and fear of being told off (Brook, 2007). This appears to outweigh their fear of pregnancy or sexually transmitted diseases. Young people who are made aware of patient confidentiality are more likely to approach the nurse for health or contraceptive advice therefore do not be judgemental when approached by an adolescent.

Adolescents do not usually welcome unsolicited health advice. This applies to all areas of health, but in practice relates especially to lifestyle, including smoking, alcohol intake, poor diet and sexual health. However, anecdotally adolescents are happy to share information about their lifestyle, such as sexuality and smoking, when asked. The following scenario offers a strategy for offering advice.

Scenario 9

Peter is a 17-year-old who attends a new patient health check accompanied by his mother. The health check comprises past medical history, present health complaints, family history, lifestyle and immunisation status. The nurse has directed the consultation to Peter, who defers to his mother when he does not know the answer. The history complete, it is time for the height and weight.

Nurse: 'I'd like to check your height and weight please. Can you take off your shoes and coat and pop next door with me?'

Peter follows the nurse.

Nurse [while weighing Peter]: 'You are 60kg. That's quite light. What did you have for breakfast?'

Peter: 'Nothing. I don't have time for breakfast.' [This contradicts the healthy diet that mum described]

Nurse briefly discusses benefits of breakfast. Moves onto measuring height.

Nurse: 'Do you have a girlfriend?'

Peter: 'Yes'

Nurse: 'I need to ask you a difficult question that I ask all people of your age. Have you ever had unprotected sex?'

Peter: 'Only once. I use protection now.'

> Nurse: 'Have you heard of chlamydia? There is a test you can send off confidentially. If you want one you can either take it now, come back when your mum isn't here, or access it from the internet.'
>
> Peter: 'I'll come back for it, thanks.'
>
> Peter and the nurse return to consulting room, where the nurse records the height and weight. There is nothing of note to share with mum, so the nurse thanks them for attending and shows them out. She then documents on the screen that Peter has been offered a chlamydia check.

In this case, the nurse used the opportunity of being alone with the adolescent to ask him personal questions when out of a parent's hearing. It is essential to be sensitive to each individual, emphasise confidentiality and let them know they can attend on their own if they wish.

Use of text messaging

Text messaging allows young people access to information or discussion about their health problems without face-to-face contact (RCN, 2006). This is a valuable means of contact for young or vulnerable people who would not usually attend a general practice surgery. There are several ways to use the messaging service, but the personal response is most relevant to practice nurses. The young person initiates the call and the nurse responds to a specific question about personal health. It can lead to a consultation or referral to another agency. It is important however to ensure the benefit to the young person outweighs the risk. If considering using this method of communication and consultation the nurse must:

- Ensure there is an up-to-date organisational confidentiality policy
- Establish client demand through a needs assessment
- Have procedures in place for child protection
- Have the resources to handle a number of texts
- Consider how and when texts will be received.
- Agree audit, review and monitoring of the service

All messages must be documented in the patient records and deleted from the receiving handset to maintain confidentiality (RCN, 2006).

E-mail

E-mail has the potential to facilitate and supplement face-to-face consultations with health professionals (Mehta and Chalhoub, 2006). Although young people are often reluctant to discuss their health problems, they readily express their concerns by e-mail, displaying high levels of directness, particularly in relation to potentially sensitive or embarrassing topics. This could be an effective method of engaging with this age group, although issues of confidentiality and documentation have yet to be addressed. Advantages and disadvantages of e-mail consultations are listed in *Box 5.2*.

A study by Moreno et al (2009) noted that many adolescents currently access healthcare information via the internet. They also reported that healthcare systems that provide online information and offer individualised advice and information tend to be more accurate than that generated by generic internet search engines. E-mail should not be a substitute for face-to-face consultations but is ideal for short questions, brief updates and follow-ups, and can be used to supplement the traditional consultation, as demonstrated in scenario 10.

Box 5.2 Advantages and disadvantages of e-mail
for consulting with young people

Advantages
1. E-mail is useful for sending links to websites and forwarding electronic leaflets.
2. When used as an adjunct to face-to face consultations, it can be used to iron out any potential misunderstandings and reinforce the important points of a previous discussion.
3. E-mail communication is cheap and quick.
4. Both the young person and the nurse can request and respond at a convenient time. Information can be filed away. The hard copy improves accurate record keeping.
5. Once trust has been established the patient may say things more openly in face-to-face consultations.

Disadvantages
1. Technical risks of e-mail include destruction of data by an electronic virus, or technical failure, and interruption of e-mail.
2. Confidentiality cannot be assured.
3. Email is not appropriate for urgent communication as the nurse could be on annual leave and not respond to the query.
4. There is the potential for over-familiarity.
5. Non-verbal communication cues are lost.

Scenario 10

Emma attended for emergency contraception. The nurse took a history, ensured there were no contraindications to the pill, counselled Emma about side-effects and generated a prescription for Levonelle. This method of emergency contraception is not 100% effective and women are asked to contact the surgery if their next period is late. The nurse asked Emma to e-mail her when she started her next period. Ten days later she received an e-mail: 'Started period today. What a relief. Emma.' The nurse was able to add this to the patient record to complete the documentation.

When considering e-mail as a method of consultation, ensure there are strict protocols and a predefined e-mail account. Use an out-of-office automatic response when away, with information of how the patient can access immediate advice. Raise the concept of e-mail consultations during a practice meeting, thus placing the responsibility for organising it with the practice manager and/or employer.

Box 5.3 offers tips for consulting with adolescents.

Box 5.3. Tips for consulting with adolescents

Do not:
- Patronise
- Be judgemental
- Appear superior
- Give unsolicited health advice.

Do:
- Offer the opportunity to see the young person without a parent
- Listen
- Reinforce confidentiality
- Give time, sympathy, respect and information
- Allow friends to support the patient during a consultation
- Signpost to relevant websites.

Minority groups and children with special needs

Young gypsies and travellers may be excluded from drugs and sex-awareness sessions at school. In some instances education in these areas is considered inappropriate by parents as they feel that awareness of these topics may lead to risk-taking behaviour. Some younger generations would not normally be expected to discuss gender or sex issues with the older generation, and would not normally get sex education from their parents. They may feel very uncomfortable in any situation where they would be expected to discuss these issues.

Disabled children and young people in Wales were asked about the services they use (Turner, 2003). A key theme that cut across all ages and abilities was the desire to be treated as an individual and be treated the same as any other child or young person. Children like to be spoken to directly and allowed to ask questions. They also appreciate small gestures such as stickers, smiles and jokes. One comment made about a GP practice was: '*...I have to wait a long time in the waiting room which is very noisy and I don't like the noise and all the people talking*'.

Children like to see the same person at every visit and be given information they understand. Consultations with minority group children should include all the consultation skills discussed previously, including tact and sensitivity. Issues relating to lesbian, gay, bisexual and transgender are discussed in Chapter 7.

Special needs encompass mild to profound learning difficulties, including autism, cerebral palsy and Downs's syndrome. The level of special needs will change throughout the child's development and nurses need to understand the implications of a child's diagnosis. A child's perception and responses is often heightened in these cases therefore patience is essential. The alternative consultation skills discussed in Chapter 6 are also relevant when working with children. Parents know their children well, so take the cues from them.

Summary

Consulting with children and adolescents can be a challenge at times. It can also be rewarding, especially when there is a good rapport and the young person trusts the nurse. It is essential to treat the child as an individual and stress confidentiality. Take time to read about the legal aspects of children consent to ensure safe practice. Consider ways to engage the young person in their care or management plan. Be friendly but not patronising, and be patient but firm.

Key points

- Involve children in their care when possible
- Respect their confidentiality
- Respect their views about health
- Treat all children and young people as individuals

Beauchamp T, Childress J (2001) *Principles of Biomedical Ethics* 5th edn. Oxford University Press, New York,

Brook (2007) *Brook's position on confidentiality*. www.brook.org.uk/content/M6_4_ confidentiality.asp

Directgov (2009) *Parental rights and responsibilities*. www.direct.gov.uk.en/...DG_4002954 accessed 28/2//2009

Department of Health (2001) *Seeking consent: working with children*. DH, London

Gregory S, Richards S (2006) Consultations with children. *Practice Nurse* **31**(9): 13–6

Martenson EK, Fagerskiold AM (2008) A review of children's decision-making competence in health care. *Journal of Clinical Nursing* **17**(23): 3131–41

Mehta S, Chalhoub N (2006) Email for your thoughts. *Child and Adolescent Mental Health* 11(3): 168–70

Moreno MA, Raiston JD, Grossman DC (2009) Adolescent Access to Online Health Services: perils and promise. *Journal of Adolescent Health* **44**(3): 244–51

Nursing and Midwifery Council (2008) *The Code. Standards of conduct, performance and ethics for nurses and midwives*. NMC, London

Robinson A (2008) Communicating with adolescents. *BMJ Learning*. www.learning.bmj. com. accessed 11/10/2008

Royal College of Nursing (2006) *Use of text messaging services. Guidance for nurses working with children and young people*. RCN, London

Turner C (2003) *Are you listening? What disabled children and young people in Wales think about the services they use. A consultation to inform the children and young people's National Service Framework*. The Welsh Assembly Government, Wales

Resources

Every Child Matters: www.everychildmatters.gov.uk

Department of Health: www.dh.gov.uk

M.E.N.D: www.nationalobesityforum.org.uk

Child Mental Health Centre: www.childmentalhealthcentre.org.uk

The Mental Health Foundation: www.mentalhealth.org.uk

Young Minds: www.youngminds.org.uk

Josef Rowntree Foundation: www.jrf.org.uk

CHAPTER 6

Patients with disabilities

Nurses must be aware of Section 21 of the Disability Discrimination Act 1995 to ensure that services are accessible to disabled people. The term disability refers to a range of conditions, including physical or mental impairment, and hearing or visual loss. The nurse will see patients with some of these conditions at some time during her working week, and needs the skills to manage the consultations with professionalism. The most significant barrier cited by the majority of disabled people is that of inappropriate staff attitudes and behaviours (Department of Health, 1999). This chapter aims to make nurses aware of consultation skills that can help redress these attitudes.

The consultation

People with a disability prefer to be seen for their individuality, not their disability. Effective and sensitive communication is an essential basic nursing skill — it is acceptable to ask courteous questions about a person's disability, or for example ask a patient with a speech impediment to repeat themselves if they are unclear. Advice and explanations should be comprehensible to patients, their relatives and carers.

The General Medical Council (GMC) (2008) offers practical tips and information for consulting with patients with a disability

- Arrange an extended appointment time for people with communication and/or physical difficulties
- Ensure that a patient's requirements are recorded on their records, for example requiring an interpreter or if a wheelchair user
- Provide interpreter services and induction loops wherever possible
- Undertake the consultation in a suitable location when necessary, for example if the patient has mobility problems
- Explain or confirm the reason for the visit, and reassure the patient.

Physical disabilities

A physical disability might be short-term, for example a broken leg or arm, or be a long-term chronic condition, for example arthritis or amputation. The most common physical disabilities that nurses are likely to encounter are patients who are wheelchair users.

The environment

The nurse should greet the patient and guide them to the prepared room where obstacles should have been removed. The environment must be adapted to allow the wheelchair user access to the consulting room. Move the furniture, such as a chair or trolley, before the patient enters the room.

Some patients will be manual wheelchair users, propelled by themselves or a companion, while others are independently mobile with an electrically operated chair. Some may require assistance, and others may feel patronised by the offer of help. It is therefore important to ascertain each person's independence. Do not forget the carer and invite the companion to be seated. The companion is not only an escort for the patient, but can be a resource for further reassurance and support.

Some consultations can take place with the patient in their chair, for example, for hypertension monitoring or health promotion advice. However, physical examinations are more difficult when carried out in a chair, and the environment must be accessible for any procedure. The Department of Health policy and guidance on disability document (DH, 1999) noted that many patients expressed their surprise that for consultations which require physical examination, they were regularly manhandled on to fixed examination couches instead of being allowed to transfer from their own wheelchairs to variable height couches. Ideally cot sides would be available for couches to provide security, as patients may have poor spatial awareness and fear falling off. If these are not available, reassure the patient at all times.

The following scenario considers the practical aspects relating to smear taking with a severely physically disabled woman.

Scenario 1

Vera is a 54-year-old woman wheelchair user who has advanced multiple sclerosis. She attended for her routine cervical smear, accompanied by her husband Bill, who is also her carer. Vera was embarrassed about having the smear because she also suffered from urinary incontinence and wore incontinence pads.

Bill assisted Vera to remove her underclothes and transfer to the couch. This protected her from the risk of manual handling injury as Bill and Vera had their own routine. Once Bill had assisted Vera he then waited outside the room while the smear was taken.

The nurse managed to visualise the cervix and take the smear unaided. If assistance had been required, she could have asked a female colleague to support Vera's legs. Following the smear, the nurse washed and dried Vera's skin and applied a clean incontinence pad and underwear. Bill then assisted Vera back into her chair.

Implications for practice
The practice was a purpose built building, designed to allow wheelchair access throughout the building. The couches were bought with accessibility in mind. Without this facility Vera would have required a home visit for this procedure, which would have been an unsuitable venue. All the examination couches in the practice were electrically operated, so could be lowered to the correct height for chair to bed transfer, to enable patients to be fully examined when required.

Reflection
Vera made an informed decision to have her smear taken, despite her disability. The nurse was aware of the disability and had made provision for the extra time and assistance required. Allowing Bill to assist Vera empowered the couple to continue their usual transfer routine, following patient-centred care. The nurse was professional, recognising Vera's anxieties and reassuring her throughout the procedure.

This scenario can be transferred to other procedures. Privacy, independence and patient autonomy must be respected at all times. Ask the patient how they wish to be assisted — many wheelchair users are independent and prefer to transfer themselves if the couch height is flexible. Do not move any mobility aid, whether wheelchair, crutches or walking stick, out of the user's reach.

Each patient is an individual, so when consulting patients with a physical disability consider their personal needs. Ask the unaccompanied wheelchair users whether or not they require help to remove clothing or transfer to the couch. They do not wish to be patronised — they are just people who are wheelchair users.

Scenario 2

Mr P is a 56-year-old man who attends for his annual diabetic review. He has a degree of osteoarthritis in his hips and knees and walks with the aid of a stick. The nurse has been seeing Mr P for the past three years and feels her heart sink when she sees him. However she hopes her smile meets her eyes and greets him.

Nurse: 'Hello, Mr P. Isn't it a lovely day?'

Mr P agrees. He sits down and the nurse discusses the blood results, which are not on target, and indicate poor blood sugar control.

Nurse: 'Your blood sugars are still too high, Mr P. Should we check your weight and see if there is any change since the last visit?'

Mr P: 'I've been trying, nurse. I'm only eating salad.'

Nurse: 'I'm sorry, Mr P. You've put on a little more weight. You are now 164kg. I'd like to check your foot pulses. You'll need to remove your shoes and socks and hop onto the bed.'

Mr P struggles to reach his feet, so the nurse assists him to remove his footwear. She lowers the couch to enable Mr P to sit on the side and supports his legs when he tries to lift them onto the couch. She raises the height of the couch and is then in the optimum position to check the foot pulses and examine the feet, without damaging her own back.

The nurse then reverses the process and assists Mr P back to the chair. She proceeds to discuss his diet and exercise habits, being sympathetic to the joint pains, but trying to reinforce previous messages of weight loss being beneficial to the joints.

The reader is probably familiar with this scenario. This is a challenging consultation. Even with the best consultation skills in the world, Mr P is difficult to motivate and is in a spiral of obesity with associated co-morbidity that will most likely deteriorate. In this situation the nurse must maintain her professional demeanour and continue to offer advice and support. Perhaps Mr P is really only eating salad, therefore the nurse must ascertain that all other avenues be addressed, including referral for medication, or a dietician for further diet advice. Physical disability can often lead to further morbidity, so the nurse needs to utilise her active listening skills and be an advocate for the patient if he wishes medication but the doctor is reluctant to prescribe. Having tried all the standard weight management options, Mr P would be a candidate for bariatric surgery. During the consultation the nurse could inform Mr P of all the options and signpost him to the appropriate doctor for action.

There are many patients with varying degrees of physical disability. Some patients are reliant on walking aids or a wheelchair. The nurse must use her skills to keep the patients as mobile as possible and reduce the risks of further morbidity. It is essential that the nurse has the skills to anticipate patient requirements during the consultation to reduce patient embarrassment by being alert to non-verbal cues, and allowing a partner to assist wherever appropriate.

Learning disabilities (intellectual disabilities)

A learning disability is a significantly reduced ability to understand new or complex information or learn new skills (impaired intelligence), with a reduced ability to cope independently (impaired social functioning), which started before adulthood, with a lasting effect on development (DH, 2009) The disability may be mild, moderate, severe or profound. Those with a mild disability may have higher levels of independence, whilst those with a profound disability may be cared for in special units, or may be cared for by their family. Practices are likely to have several patients with a learning disability in their population, and nurses need the consultation skills to offer these patients equitable care.

Informed consent

The area of informed consent poses many dilemmas for practice nurses. The Mental Capacity Act 2005 states that the presence of a learning disability must not lead to a presumed inability to consent to all interventions (DH, 2007). Although a patient with a learning disability may consent to a procedure, is it really an informed decision, or are they doing what you want them to do?

Consent for patients with learning disabilities who are regarded as unable to give valid consent is usually sought from a third party. Relatives, carers or friends may be able to give an indication of the patient's wishes (Reeves and Orford, 2002), but are unable to give consent on the patient's behalf. Nurses must act in the patient's best interests at all times. On some occasions the nurse might administer an injection, such as the annual flu injection, without patient consent.

The NMC Code (2008) states that:

'You must be aware of the legislation regarding mental capacity, ensuring that people who lack capacity remain at the centre of decision making and are fully safeguarded.'

A person is more likely to give valid consent if the explanation is appropriate to the level of his/her assessed ability. Nurses should utilise the expertise of their learning disability nurse colleagues to ensure patients with limited mental competence receive quality care as these nurses have the skills and tools to help the patient understand a procedure. Information is put into easier-to-read formats to help those with a learning disability understand; this includes the use of pictures and simple language.

The three main areas of concern regarding consent for practice nurses are immunisation, contraception and cervical cytology. These are invasive procedures that may be difficult to explain in a language the patient understands. Many of the patients who live in the community will have a key worker or family member who has a deeper understanding of the patient's mental ability. It may be necessary to defer a procedure until the key worker can work with the patient, using appropriate material to help gain an informed decision or consent.

Communication

Learning-disabled patients are reported to have difficulty in healthcare consultations due to inappropriate communication, including staff who talked too loudly or spoke as if the patients were children (DH, 1999). Mencap (2008) suggest the best way to communicate is to pick up on non-verbal gestures, like facial expressions, grimaces, and body language. Patients with a learning disability read other peoples' body language well, so nurses should be aware of their own body language. Patients with a profound and multiple learning disability will usually have a support worker who understands the patient's communication pattern. Keep information brief and simple and avoid using jargon.

Patients with a learning disability might have trouble remembering names and faces, so it is helpful if the nurse briefly reintroduces herself at each consultation (Thacker, 2002). This will vary according to the level of disability, but anecdotally in the author's practice, patients who attend regularly for chronic disease management or for an annual review with the same nurse know their nurse's name. However, it is still helpful to remind some patients by saying something like: '*Hello Pauline. I saw you last year, do you remember me?*'.

Some patients prefer pictures and the written word above spoken language. Prepared materials exist to help patients describe symptoms and to help the nurse explain to a patient. These include explaining what will happen in an examination, such as a cervical smear. Liaise with the learning disability team for resources if these are not available in the practice. See *Figure 6.1* for examples of how pictures can be used in invitation letters. Ideally the letter would have a picture of the nurse they are to see.

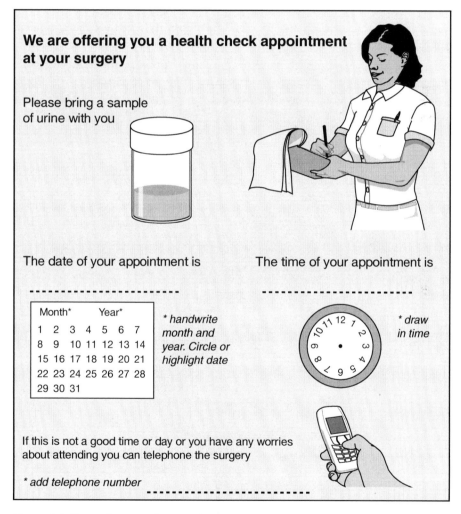

Figure 6.1 Illustrative appointment letter

Time can be a difficult concept for some people to describe. If Roger is asked how long he has had the sore on his leg, the response will often be vague. Thacker (2002) suggests linking symptoms to an 'index event' such as a key date, or to how many times have they been to bed since the problem started. Patients will often answer 'yes' if asked if they understand what has been said. It can be more helpful to invite them to say in their own words what they understand.

The consultation

Remember that people with intellectual disabilities need sufficient time to allow them to speak for themselves (Perez, 2002). If possible, tag the patient records with an alert that flags up their disability. The person making the appointment is then reminded to book a double appointment slot, preferably the first appointment of the session. Some people have difficulty waiting in a busy room and may get distressed, and/or upset other patients. *Box 6.1* lists top tips for effective consultations with a patient with learning difficulties.

Box 6.1 Tips for effective consultation

1. Ask for information prior to the appointment so the patient can think what to say
2. Enable the person to speak for themselves
3. Reassure, with positive body language
4. Assess patient's understanding and use language they understand
5. Speak to the patient, not the carer
6. Use open questions
7. Show the patient any equipment to be used
8. Ask the carer for supportive information
9. Use events when talking about time
10. Avoid using jargon
11. Smile

(adapted from Perez, 2002)

Key issues to consider during the consultation include:
- Ask the patient if they want a carer present
- Encourage and empower the person to speak for themselves. This can be difficult when protective elderly parents accompany their adult 'child'. Some carers will encourage the patient to speak, whilst others take over the consultation. This may be due to limited consultation time.
- The carer will usually be able to advise the nurse on the best way to communicate with an individual. As noted above, some patients communicate best through pictures.

- Direct questions to the patient, and not to the carer, although the patient can ask the carer for help. This will aid patient empowerment.
- Open questions will elicit more information than closed. Reword questions to see if the response is the same, and the patient has understood the question.
- Show the patient any equipment that will be used prior to use, for example the auroscope and ear irrigation machine. Also let the patient hear the noise of the machine to reassure them what to expect.
- Although the patient should be the primary speaker, it can be helpful if the carer corroborates or refutes the given information. The patient might be confused about a certain issue.
- Patients may have little or no understanding of time. Explain the use of medications in terms of events, such as: '*...use the cream before breakfast and before bed*'.
- Do not confuse the patient with medical jargon. Use simple language with those who are intellectually impaired.

Although the patient might attend for a particular reason, use this opportunity to assess their general health, including the presence of earwax, feet problems, and risk of cardiovascular disease. The scenario below is an example of a simple consultation.

Scenario 3

Ruth attended for a flu vaccination. She had mild Downs's syndrome but was anxious in a group, so was always seen in the general surgery rather than the flu clinic. The nurse gained informed consent, ensured there were no contraindications and administered the injection. Ruth then produced an empty box out of her handbag and asked for more of the same. She was asking for hydrocortisone/fungal cream.

Nurse: 'What are you using this for?'

Ruth: 'For my feet.'

Nurse checks Ruth's patient records and sees that she has had several acute prescriptions for this cream. Long-term steroid cream is not recommended and the nurse was unwilling to supply another tube without ensuring it was clinically indicated.

Nurse: 'Could you take your trainers and socks off, so I can look at your feet, please?'

Ruth removes her socks and trainers and the nurse examines her feet. There is no evidence that topical steroids are required. There is however, slight fungal infection between the toes.

Nurse: 'You do need cream for your feet, Ruth. I will get the doctor to prescribe a different cream. I will write a note for your carer, so she will know what to do. Wash your feet every day and use the cream between your toes.' [Demonstrates on herself]

A prescription is generated and signed. The nurse writes a note to the carer, explaining that steroid cream is not needed and that an anti-fungal cream is more appropriate and should be applied to clean feet 1–2 times a day. She draws a picture of a foot and a tube of cream, and draws 08:00am and 18:00pm on two clocks. This reminds Ruth when she needs to apply the cream. If she has any questions she can contact the nurse. She then documents this in the patient records.

During this consultation the nurse used simple language in short sentences, and the nurse did not consider it appropriate to explain the difference between the creams. The written note reinforced the advice and would be added to her care plan by the carer/support worker. Praise and reassurance will encourage the patient to follow instructions.

Consulting with a parent or support worker present

Patients with a learning disability may attend by themselves, with a family member, or a support worker. There are advantages and disadvantages of the patient being accompanied.

Advantages:
- Can confirm medications, current health status and symptoms
- Can recall diet and exercise pattern
- Can take home the health message and any instructions, for example if a blood test is needed
- Can supply background information where necessary

Disadvantages:
- Interrupts the nurse and/or patient
- Dominates the consultation by talking for the patient
- Manipulates the consultation
- Can be in denial of health issue.

Health issues

People with a learning disability now live to pensionable age and are therefore susceptible to the diseases of old age, including diabetes and coronary heart disease. Edwards (2007) discussed the major health issues relating to this patient group. These include obesity, which can be related to poor diet, lack of activity or some psychogenic drugs. Respiratory tract infections tend to be caused by aspiration or reflux, rather than asthma or chronic obstructive airways disease, and the nurse should advise patients to have their influenza and pneumococcal vaccines. Gastro-oesophageal reflux disease is also common but patients may not know how to describe their symptoms.

Health action plans

A health action plan is an individualised plan offering guidance to stay healthy, and aids multi-agency working. This is particularly important when a patient has several support workers to ensure the patient receives maximum health input. The plan can be shared with family, carers, support workers, and the community learning disability team. It should involve an easy-to-read format written plan for the patient. Appropriate leaflets, booked appointments and advice is also given so the patient, who can share it with the carer if he/she wishes. Table 6.1 is an example of what might be recorded after an annual review. The patient has a copy and the written plan is scanned into the patient notes as a record of the action and advice.

Table 6.1 Example of a health action plan.

Health issue	Actions needed to keep you healthy
Diabetes	Try not to eat sweets and cakes. Keep walking and swimming every week Book a blood test on ...... date
New Problem: High Blood Pressure	Take your tablets every day. Appointment booked on ..... date to see nurse for blood pressure check
Wax in right ear	Use olive oil drops 4 times a day for 4 days Appointment booked on .... date for ear irrigation
At risk of flu	Book flu injection on .... date
Plan completed by: Name: Date:	Next appointment date:

The nurse should contact the learning disability team for special concerns, such as help in gaining consent for a procedure, or for more intensive support, for example for weight management, and identify any additional support required in the patient's notes. It is important to remember that all forms of change require adjustment to routine.

Sexual health

Smear tests

It is common for women with a learning disability not to be offered a routine smear test on the assumption that they have never had sexual intercourse (NHSCSP, 2008). However this should not be assumed and furthermore the woman may have experienced sexual abuse without the carer or support worker's knowledge. The use of leaflets to reinforce the value of both smears and breast screening might improve uptake in this marginalized group of women.

Before a smear, the woman should have been prepared by the nurse and/or community learning disability nurse by explaining what a smear is and why it is needed. Adapted, easy-to-read information, a cloth model doll and DVD material can be used as preparation material. When a woman does attend for a cervical smear, ensure that an appropriate length appointment time is booked. If a support worker accompanies the woman, she might stand at the head of the bed and hold the woman's hand for reassurance. When carrying out the procedure it is important to include the following steps:

*   Reinforce the purpose of the smear
*   Ensure she has some understanding of the procedure
*   Explain what you are doing at every step
*   Show the woman the speculum and brush before use
*   Use appropriate language and pictures
*   Be patient and take each step slowly
*   If the woman resists or pushes the speculum away, stop the procedure.

Barriers to the completion of the procedure could include:

*   Lack of understanding
*   Fear
*   Previous bad experience
*   Possible sexual abuse.

It is essential to reassure the woman during the procedure and praise her when the procedure is completed. This is relevant for any procedure to both women and men. The smear result is posted to the patient's home address, although the carer may have to explain the result. In the case of an abnormal smear, the nurse is advised to liaise with her learning disability colleagues to help her explain the result to the patient and follow up procedures.

Breast examination

All women are at risk of breast cancer. In the author's community, one local learning disability team has held a series of sessions for teaching breast awareness within the practice. The practice nurse was the link between the team and the women. She explained about the sessions during the annual health checks, to prepare the women and their carers for the training. Carers were also invited to attend the teaching sessions, both to reassure the women and to assist in future breast awareness. The rapport between nurse and patient gained through regular reviews resulted in good attendance and good feedback to the team. The older women are currently being prepared for mammography using the same model.

In this context the practice nurse should use her interpersonal communication skills to develop multidisciplinary working to benefit the patients. Consultation skills are as important when dealing with colleagues and families as with patients.

Testicular self-examination

Men with a learning disability are entitled to receive care that is sensitive and effective, specifically with regard to testicular self-examination (Peate and Maloret, 2007). This is no different to the care given to all young men. A leaflet and guidance might be all a young man requires to encourage him to self examine. Testicular self-examination can be carried out independently if the man has a mild learning disability, or with assistance of another person, for example a carer or partner. In the latter case, the man must give consent for the procedure.

If the man lives within his family unit, advising the father to help teach and support his son is ideal, but will depend on their relationship.

In the author's community a local learning disability team are planning a series of sessions to teach the men about their bodies following the good evaluation of the breast awareness sessions. Practice nurses could liaise with their own teams to be involved in training, or learn from their colleagues.

Scenarios 4 and 5 incorporates issues of communication, informed consent and liaison with appropriate professionals to achieve an effective consultation.

Scenario 4

Mary and John both have mild to moderate learning disabilites. When they married in 2008, Mary attended the practice for contraception advice. The nurse was unable to discuss the implications of contraception, and asked her community learning disability (LD) colleagues for help to explain sex education and contraception.

It was important to identify contraindications to any method of contraception as Mary was taking anti-epilepsy medication that interfered with the combined oral contraception, which if taken would have been ineffective. An effective method had to be acceptable to both Mary and John.

The practice nurse liaised with her LD colleagues and explained the possible contraception options for Mary. They then used their easy-read education material and soft cloth doll to deliver sex education to Mary and John. After considering all the options, the most appropriate form of contraception was the long-acting Depovera injection. Mary continued to attend for the long acting contraception injection. She was given a card with the date of the next due injection, which she showed her support worker. She then wrote the date on Mary's calendar and reminded her the week the injection was due.

Implications for practice

Mary and John did not want children and a reliable method of contraception was essential. The practice nurse did not have the specialist skills of her LD colleague, but shared working resulted in an appropriate method being chosen.

Reflective practice

The nurse did not feel confident discussing sex education and contraception with Mary. Although Mary continued to attend for her injections, the nurse relied on her LD colleagues to assist in supporting her when Mary was due for her cervical smear. Multidisciplinary teamwork is essential to ensure patients receive the best possible care.

Scenario 5

Michael attended unaccompanied for a booked appointment with the nurse. He attended periodically for dressings to his inflamed shins, which he subconsciously scratched. There had been a two-month break since the last visit. On this occasion there was evidence of cellulitis and scratch marks with open sores to both legs.

Nurse: 'Why do you scratch your legs?'

Michael: 'Because they itch.'

Nurse: 'But when you scratch your legs they become sore.' [Points to the broken skin]

Michael: 'Yes, I know.' [Subconsciously continues to scratch]

Nurse [shows him a zinc paste bandage]: 'This will help to heal the sores.' [The rationale was to cover the legs and prevent scratching]

Michael returned for review with his support worker.

Support worker: 'Michael is upset because he can't have a bath. He feels dirty.'

Michael: 'I feel dirty.'

Nurse checks the leg and notes signs of healing.

Nurse: 'Your legs look much better today. Can I put the bandage on again? You will need these for a few weeks, but you can have a bath.'

The nurse reapplied the bandages and generated a prescription for waterproof protective leg covers. The nurse explained their application to the support worker, who helped Michael bathe.

Michael was happy with the management plan because he was able to bathe regularly. He attended regularly for dressings, although not always on the right day or at the right time. The nurses were used to him and were flexible in their approach, so he was always seen. Once the skin was clear, a moisturising cream was prescribed to prevent dry skin and recurrence of the itch/scratch cycle. This was to be applied at least twice a day. The instructions were explained to Michael and written down for him to take to his support workers. A written, timed, follow up appointment to see the nurse was made for two weeks to ensure the skin was intact.

In this case it was important to encourage Michael to continue the treatment plan — which was simple once his needs had been acknowledged. Nurses who consult with patients with a learning disability require patience, flexibility and understanding. The support worker or carer needs a clear written plan of action to enable the care to be continued at home.

Nurses must develop the consultation skills to offer patients with a learning disability equitable care. These patients have more healthcare needs than the rest of the population, and assessing cardiovascular risk factors, managing long-term conditions, and dealing with minor injuries all require special skills. Support workers are the key to maintaining the patients' adherence with treatment and attendance at appointments, therefore ensure they are kept abreast of patient management plans.

Patients who are deaf or hard of hearing

All practice populations are different, but most are likely to have some patients who are deaf or hard of hearing. This could be congenital deafness, age related or occupational. It is impossible to undertake an effective consultation if the patient cannot communicate with the nurse. Ideally, the patient notes should be tagged so that the nurse is aware that the next patient has a hearing impairment. This will prevent any embarrassment — the nurse who collects her patients from the waiting room will not overlook the one who missed their name being called by the receptionist or intercom.

Communication

Always face the patient when speaking. Note that people with a hearing loss might agree with, or accept, what has been said even if they do not fully understand the advice or instructions. This could be a habit as they do not wish to offend or frustrate the nurse.

Burke (2007) suggests improvements that can be made to reduce the awkwardness and frustration of communicating with this group of patients. These relate to:

Physical
- Make sure all your face can be seen.
- Sit at the same height as the patient and maintain eye contact.
- Do not have anything in your mouth.
- Trim a beard or moustache so it does not block the mouth (for the men!).
- Have pen and paper to hand to communicate by writing.

Environmental
- Position yourself in a good light source. This helps with seeing speech and signs.
- Try to monitor noise levels, as noise can distract understanding.

Verbal
- Some people prefer slower speech, others normal speech. Try to elicit which the patient prefers.
- Repeat or paraphrase as necessary.

Nonverbal
- Use facial expressions and gestures.
- Touch the shoulder, arm or leg to gain their attention and reassure them if they are close to you.

Box 6.2 offers some tips when speaking to someone who has a hearing impairment. A free A5 format communication tip card is available from the Royal National Institute for the Deaf (RNID).

Box 6.2 Tips when speaking to someone who is deaf
or hard of hearing

- Even if someone is wearing a hearing aid, it does not mean they can hear. Ask if they need to lip-read you.
- Make sure you have the patient's attention before speaking and maintain eye contact.
- Speak clearly but not too slowly, and do not exaggerate your lip movements.
- Use natural facial expressions and gestures, and smile.
- When you have both a hearing and deaf person in the room, do not just focus on the hearing person.
- Do not shout. It is uncomfortable for a hearing aid user and looks aggressive.
- If the patient does not understand what you say, do not keep repeating it but try saying it another way.
- Do not turn your face away from a deaf person.
- Check that the patient can follow what you are saying. Be patient and take the time to communicate properly.
- Use plain language and do not waffle. Avoid jargon and unfamiliar abbreviations.

Source: RNID (2004)

Lip reading

Everyone lip reads to some extent, especially in noisy situations. Facial movements give information to help people understand the meaning of what is being said. Many hard of hearing people also lip read. It requires a lot of skill and concentration when talking to someone who lip reads, and can sometimes be tiring. Many words look similar on the lips, and some sounds are pronounced at the back of the throat and have no visible lip shape. *Box 6.3* lists tips to help the lip reader.

The nurse should note that once a patient removes their hearing aid/s, they are suddenly bereft and isolated. Therefore it is essential to explain any procedure before removing the aids and allow the patient to lip read during the consultation. Refer to scenario 6.

Box 6.3 Tips to help the lip reader

- Ask the patient if they can lip read before starting the conversation.
- Try and find the quietest place possible for a conversation.
- Ask the patient to stand or sit facing the light, and avoid shadows.
- Sit or stand on the same level and between three and six feet from the patient.
- The patient should not feel embarrassed about asking for things to be repeated or asking for something to be said in a different way.
- The patient needs to watch the nurse's whole face, not only the lips. Facial expressions and gestures tell a lot about what is being said.
- Keep a pen and paper handy.
- Stop as soon as something is missed, and repeat what was said

It is common for patients to attend for ear irrigation before attending a hearing clinic. Allowing the patient to lip read is often necessary in these circumstances.

Source: RNID (2004)

Sign language

The most significant barrier in effectively accessing and using health service provision for people whose first language is sign language was inappropriate and ineffective communication (Freeney et al, 1999). It is therefore a misconception that offering written information to deaf people is adequate for informed consent.

The most significant barrier for sign language users is the absence of an interpreter or communication support. These patients require a longer

---

Scenario 6

Mr E attends for ear irrigation. The nurse welcomes him, notes that he wears bilateral hearing aids, invites him to be seated and clarifies the reason for the consultation.

Nurse: 'It's nice to see you again, Mr E. What can I do for you today?'

Mr E: 'It's my ears, nurse. I've got to go for a new mould next week.'

Patient shows nurse the letter from the clinic asking him to have his ears checked prior to the appointment.

Nurse: 'I'll check your ears first if that's alright.'

Mr E [taking his aids out]: 'I won't hear a word you say now.'

Nurse faces Mr E and explains that she will now look in his ears. Mr E nods to express his understanding. The nurse looks in both ears with the otoscope and sees the drums are clear. She then faces Mr E and hands him his aids.

Mr E replaces hearing aids and switches them on.

Nurse: 'Your ears are fine, Mr E. There is no wax in them, so you should have no problems with the moulds.'

Mr E: 'Thank you, nurse. Goodbye.'

The nurse records in the patient notes that the drums were visible and that irrigation was not performed.

---

time to assimilate explanations. Face the patient in good light while speaking, and explain all procedures before and during the event.

Where a patient uses a paid interpreter it is essential that the patient is seen on time, as the interpreter is unlikely to be able to stay if it means missing a later engagement.

Finally, ensure that the patient with a hearing impairment has fully understood any explanation, including medications and review dates before they leave the consulting room.

Loop induction system

Ask yourself the following questions: is there a portable loop induction system for use in consultations? Where is it? How does it work?

An induction loop is a cable that encloses the audience area. It connects to a loop amplifier that gets its signal from a microphone placed in front of the person speaking. It can also get a signal from a direct connection such as a sound system. The resulting electric current in the loop produces a magnetic field corresponding to the speaker's voice. A loop system can help the patient to hear sound more clearly if they use a hearing aid with a 'T' setting or loop listener because it helps to reduce background noise. Induction loops and infrared systems reduce the effect of background noise so deaf people can hear sound more clearly.

The deaf person uses a receiver that converts the signal back to sound. With loop systems, this is usually their hearing aid. Both systems allow users to hear from anywhere covered by the system. The sound that people hear without a receiver is unaffected.

Portable loops are (usually) designed to cover a small area and can be packed away after use. They are useful when a permanent system is not needed, or if needed in different rooms.

Anyone within the area of the loop who is wearing a hearing aid switched to the 'T' setting, or a loop listening aid, can pick up sound from the loop. Users may need to adjust their own hearing aids for volume. Receivers can be supplied to anyone who does not have a suitable hearing aid. It is not usually feasible to use a magnetic induction to convey stereo sound unless someone is wearing very small loops worn at each ear (known as ear hooks).

Text messaging

A mobile phone can be used to send SMS text messages as reminders for appointments, or when the patient has a query. Although there will be few practices currently using this service, it is a method of communication that deserves investigation.

Ethnic minority patients

It was reported that those from minority ethnic backgrounds are likely to be doubly disadvantaged in accessing health services and related information, with approximately 100 000 deaf people in the UK belonging to ethnic minority groups who cannot speak or understand fluent English (Freeney et al, 1999). This is discussed in more detail in Chapter 9. The need for deafness awareness has been recognised and publicised (Harrison, 2008).

Formal training in deaf awareness and practical communication skills is needed in all general practices.

Patients who are blind or visually impaired

There are around two million people in the UK with a sight problem. This means that while wearing glasses they are still unable to recognise someone across the road or have difficulty reading newsprint. Among these two million people, over 370 000 are registered as blind or partially sighted. Only a small percentage of people who are registered blind or partially sighted can see nothing at all (Action for Blind People et al, 2009). There could be an additional 20% who are eligible for registration but have not yet done so (RNIB, 2008). Blurred vision, distortions or defects in the visual field are also included in the term visual defect.

Not all patients will carry a white stick. Some will be visually impaired but unaccompanied. Others will have a companion who guides them. Always consider confidentiality when a patient is accompanied. Ask the patient if they wish to be seen alone, and respect whatever decision they make.

The following tips might be helpful when you see a visually impaired patient:
- Introduce yourself and make sure the person knows you are speaking to them
- Talk directly to them and not through a third party
- If you are going to guide them, let them take your arm, do not grab theirs
- Mention any potential hazards that lie ahead and say where they are
- If you are guiding someone into a seat, place their hand on the back of the seat before they sit down, so they can orientate themselves
- Do not walk away without saying you are leaving

The biggest difficulty expressed by blind and visually impaired patients during a consultation is not knowing what was happening to them whilst being examined (DH, 1999). Therefore it is important that the patient knows exactly what their consultation will entail (Action for Blind People et al, 2009). Best practice is to introduce yourself and anyone else in the room, for example a GP registrar; use the patient's name, and explain every stage of the consultation so that there are no surprises, especially where physical contact is required.

A visually impaired person does not see but 'feels' the world through touch, sense and hearing. The tone of voice can convey many messages, including frustration and boredom.

Some visually impaired people find conversation difficult. Without eye contact and awareness of body language it can be hard to connect with other people. A light touch on the arm will indicate to them that they are being spoken to. Before you move away, say that you are about to leave. Everyone feels foolish talking to an empty space. Check that the patient is comfortable with any lighting change, for example if you need brighter light to examine a minor injury. See scenario 7.

Print

Many people with low vision can read standard print if it is well designed. They may also use magnification or certain lighting to improve readability. Large and giant print is essential for many blind and partially sighted people. No single size is suitable for everyone. Large print is usually in the range of 16 to 22 point. Giant print uses fonts that are 24 point plus. Bear this in mind when offering literature. If you are downloading information leaflets from the internet, try to increase font size.

It is wrong to assume that all patients will have someone to open and read their letters. It might be more appropriate to telephone the patient, discuss what is required and make the convenient appointment. Action for Blind People et al (2009) cite an example of a patient missing appointments because she was not quick enough to get help to read her letters.

This reinforces the need to tag patient records with a note of a person's disability to prevent this type of scenario. See scenario 8.

Medication and information for aftercare

Nurses are reminded to ensure that patients know how to take their medication and/or care for wounds (Action for Blind People et al, 2009). When antibiotics are prescribed for an infected wound, it is essential to be quite clear with the instructions as not all patients understand how to follow instructions on the packet.

As the medication literature is usually in very small print it is important to explain to the patient potential side-effects. Make any follow-up appointment while the patient is in the room, and ask them to repeat what has been said to ensure they have understood. Reinforce this with a written appointment card using large print as a reminder.

Guide dogs

Some patients will attend with their guide dog. There is no reason why this should not be allowed, unless an invasive procedure such as a minor operation

Scenario 7

Mr R attended for his regular Zoladex injection. He was accompanied by his wife.

Nurse: 'Hello, Mr R, Mrs R. Please take a seat.' [Guides Mr R to the seat, places his hands on the arms and waits until he is seated.]

Nurse: 'What are we doing today?' [Confirming that the patient is expecting his injection.]

Mr R: 'It's that nasty injection again.'

The nurse has prepared for this consultation and has the Zoladex in her room. She prepares the injection, considering all aspects of infection control.

Nurse: 'Where will you be most comfortable? Lying on the bed or sitting in the chair?' [Considers patient comfort.]

Mr R: 'I usually sit in the chair, if that's alright with you?'

Nurse: 'That's fine. If you could just undo your trousers for me.'

Allows patient to partially undress in privacy.

Nurse: 'I am just going to wash my hands.' [Explains to patient.]

Nurse: 'OK. I've got the injection here. Are you ready?' [Prepares patient.]

Mr R nods.

Nurse: 'You'll feel a sharp scratch now.' [Gives warning of needle being inserted.]

Nurse concludes the consultation by clearing away the equipment, washing her hands and completing the relevant documentation. At all stages she kept Mr R informed about where she was, and what she was going to do.

is planned. It is wise not to fuss the dog without the prior permission of the owner. A nurse who has an allergy to, or fear of, dogs will need to liaise with a colleague, who might be able to assist in the consultation.

Scenario 8

Mr W is due for a coronary heart disease review. The nurse has trawled the list of non-attendees and noted he had not been reviewed for over a year. She sent a standard letter, requesting Mr W to book in for a blood test and then to see her the following week. The nurse wondered why Mr W failed to attend either appointment.

Options:
1.   He had left the area
2.   He was on holiday
3.   The appointment was inconvenient
4.   He could not read the letter.

Summary

Nurses are likely to encounter patients with a disability in their practice. Always face the patient and not the computer when talking. Ask them to repeat what has been said to ensure they have understood. Be aware that some people have both visual and hearing problems, and that a physical disability does not preclude a visual loss.

Key points

*   Be aware of 'who' the next patient is, including the support they require
*   Action from the nurse is required to make the appointment outcome a success
*   Continuity of care can maintain or improve quality of life.

Action for Blind People, The Guide Dogs for the Blind and Royal Institute for the Blind (2009) *Patient focus. How to provide a good service to blind and partially sighted people*. RNIB, London

Burke J (2007) *Hearing Loss – Communicate with Deaf or Hard of Hearing People*. Deafness. www.deafness.about.com/od/heari... accessed 13/10/2008

Department of Health (1999) *Working in partnership to implement section 21 of the Disability Discrimination Act 1995 across the National Health Service*. DH, London

Department of Health (2007) *Mental Capacity Act 2005*. DH, London

Department of Health (2009) *Valuing People: a new three year strategy for people with a learning disability*. DH, London

Edwards M (2007) Caring for patients with a learning disability. *Practice Nurse* **34**(3): 38–41

Freeney M, Cook R, Hale B, Duckworth S (1999) *Working in partnership to implement section 21 of the Disability Discrimination Act 1995 across the National Health Service*. DoH, London

General Medical Council (2008) *Disability*. www.gmc-uk.org/.../disability accessed 8/1/2009

Harrison E (2008) Deafness awareness straining is vital. *Independent Nurse* **3 Nov:** 17

Mencap (2008) *Checklist summary*. www.mencap.org.uk/page.as... accessed 21/12/2008

NHS Cancer Screening Programmes (2008) *NHS Cervical Screening Programme*. www.cancerscreening.nhs.uk/cervical accessed 25/1/2009

Nursing and Midwifery Council (2008) *The Code. Standards of conduct, performance and ethics for nurses and midwives*. NMC, London

Peate I, Maloret P (2007) Testicular self-examination: the person with learning disabilities. *British Journal of Nursing* **16**(15): 931–5

Perez W (2002) *Top ten tips for effective consultation*. www.intellectualdisability.info/values/top_ten_tips.htm accessed 20/10/2008

Reeves M, Orford J (2002) *Fundamental Aspects of Legal, Ethical and Professional Issues in Nursing*. Quay Books, Wilts

RNIB (2008) *About sight loss - changing the way we think about blindness*. www.rnib.org.uk accessed 21/12/2008

Royal National Institute for the Deaf (2004) *Communication tips* (card). RNID, London

Thacker A (2002) *Clinical Communication*. www.intellectualdisability.info/.../clin_com accessed 21/12 2008

Resources

Action for Blind People: www.afbp.org

Deafblind UK: www.deafblind.org.uk

Just Advocacy: www.justadvocacy.org.uk

Mencap: www.mencap.org.uk

NHS Cancer Screening Programmes: www.cancerscreening.nhs.uk

RNIB: www.rnib.org.uk

RNID: www.rnid.org.uk

Valuing People: www.valuingpeople.gov.uk

CHAPTER 7

Sexual orientation

Sexual orientation sometimes raises connotations of the stereotypical butch women and effeminate men. However, in reality it is not always possible to assess someone's sexuality on first meeting. And does it matter? All patients are entitled to be treated in the same manner. Providing equitable health services demands that provision is culturally appropriate, sensitive and inclusive. This is made clear in the Equality Act (Sexual Orientation) Regulations 2007 which states that lesbian, gay, bisexual and transgender (LGBT) people cannot be refused treatments that would be offered to anyone else.

Harassment can occur if a person's dignity is violated or an intimidating, hostile, degrading, humiliating or offensive environment is created (General Medical Council, 2008). This relates to any patient, but in this chapter is used in the context of sexual orientation. Research from Stonewall (2006a) suggests that the gay population do not receive the same health care and are stigmatised due to their sexuality. It is recognised that some healthcare workers are uncomfortable providing services to LGBT patients (Neville and Henrickson, 2006). This chapter aims to highlight good practice consultation skills which can be used to improve the health of this practice population.

Comments and quotes in the text include data from two small groups of homosexual men and women surveyed by the author in March 2009. The author undertook an informal survery of homosexual men and women introduced by mutual friends. A total of 14 offered comments on their health care.

Disclosure

It is estimated that 5–7% of the population are LGBT, although exact figures are unknown (Stonewall, 2006b). There are conflicting studies on the experiences of lesbian women. A literature review by Phillips-Angeles et al (2004) found healthcare providers to be judgmental, non–supportive and negative when a lesbian's sexual orientation was known. This included the disturbing fact that many homosexual women decide to discontinue care because of the negative experiences they encounter after disclosure. It can also be assumed that homosexual and bisexual men encounter similar experiences. However another study found that lesbians who disclose their sexual orientation to their provider reported increased comfort, better communication and had a greater likelihood of seeking health services (Steele et al, 2006). Although these studies are contradictory, the author's experiences suggest that LGBTs are often loth to disclose their sexuality to health professionals.

Although the following relates to doctors (Stonewall/GMC, 2008), the same issues can be transferred to practice nurses and should be considered during a consultation. Patients reported that doctors:

- Fail to examine or respond to a patient properly, for example they have not been willing to offer a smear test to a lesbian woman;
- Told others they are gay, when this had nothing to do with their treatment.

Relevant guidance from the Royal College of Nursing and Unison (2004) is summarised in *Box 7.1*.

Box 7.1 Guidance on homosexual and transgender service users

- Be aware that you may have homosexual and transgender service users, even if you do not know who they are.
- Be sensitive about the way you request information from service users, using language that is inclusive and gender neutral.
- Make it safe for same sex partners and family members to be open about their relationships if they want to so they can be supported during illness or crisis.
- Respect privacy and confidentiality.
- If necessary, provide LBGT service users and their families with details of where to get further, specialist support, advice and information.

Confidentiality, documentation and inclusiveness

Healthcare workers should never make a record of a service user's sexual orientation without their previous permission (RCN and Unison, 2004). Nurses should give LGBT patients opportunities for disclosure as well as seeking permission to pass that information to healthcare colleagues who may be involved in their care. This saves LGBT patients the additional stress of explaining their situation when seeing another member of the team (Neville and Henrickson, 2006).

Of the eight gay men in one of the groups surveyed by the author in March 2009, only three are open and honest about their sexual orientation to their GP. Most are still frightened that they may get 'victimised' if they were open about their sexuality. One of the big concerns of one survey participant was that somehow his sexuality would be on his medical records and that this information might be communicated to a third party, for example, if he applied for life insurance or had a medical for a new job.

Do not make assumptions about a person's sexuality. In a study by Neville and Henrickson (2006), approximately three quarters of respondents reported that their healthcare provider 'always' or 'usually' presumed that they were heterosexual unless told otherwise. Consider scenario 1 below. Inclusiveness does not just mean not making assumptions about a person's sexual orientation, but making sure that all patients are getting the correct treatment and are being included into all relevant screening programmes.

Homosexual couples considering parenting can be advised in much the same way as all other couples, however attention to the role of the non-biological parent as an equal parent is essential. Due consideration may be given to the sensitivity of the legal status of homosexual relationships. This may be relevant for consent if the non-biologic parent brings a child for immunisation (see Chapter 3). Rather than assume a baby has a 'daddy' or a 'mummy' — it is good practice to use the term 'parent'.

Scenario 1

Sally visited the doctor at her partner's insistence because she had been having a lingering cough for several weeks. The doctor was a young female in her late 20s.

Sally explained to the doctor that her partner had asked her to come to the surgery about her coughing. When the doctor next referred to Sally's partner, she referred to a 'he'. Sally had to explain to the doctor that her partner was a 'she', putting both the doctor and Sally in an embarrassing situation.

Reflection
This situation could have been avoided if the doctor had referred to Sally's partner neutrally instead of assuming it would be a male partner. It would then have been up to Sally to decide if she wanted to reveal her partner's sex to the doctor

---

Transgender

Transgender is the broad term used to include transvestites, transgender and transsexual people. Transgender is reported to be a birth condition and not a state of mind (Transgender Zone, 2009). These people have complex gender identities, and can move from one category to another over time (Whittle et al, 2007). The true number of transgender people in the UK is unknown, but was estimated to be about 5000 in 2007. It is important to be aware that transgender people may be lesbian, bisexual, gay or heterosexual.

Gender identity disorders in children and adolescents are rare and complex conditions, sometimes with genetic conditions, which are often associated with emotional and behavioural difficulties (Asscheman et al, 1989).

In one study, 17% of respondents had experienced a doctor or nurse who did not approve of gender reassignment and refused their services, while 23% felt that being transgender affected the way they were treated by healthcare professionals (Whittle et al, 2007).

There are many studies into the effects of transgender hormonal treatment including depression, increased risk of suicide, cardiovascular disease and thrombotic events, weight gain and acne. Gender awareness would help the nurse advise the patient sensitively and appropriately.

Issues that might require sensitive handling during consultations include:

- Male-to-female surgical reassignment, when promoting sexual health, contraception or cervical cytology.
- Female-to-male reassignment if the man is still registered as woman at the health authority and is called for a cervical smear.
- Empathy if the patient is being bullied or harassed.
- Explaining the rationale for monitoring weight and cardiovascular disease risk.

Privacy, confidentiality and individualised care should be the accepted norm. Training in transgender health would enable the nurse to develop his/her skills to offer transgender patients the right to be treated as a member of their new gender (Whittle et al, 2007).

Sexual health

A 2007 survey of over 6000 homosexual women highlighted that less than half of homosexual and bisexual women have ever been screened for sexually transmitted diseases (Stonewall, 2008). Of these, 15% over the age of 25 years have never had a cervical smear test, compared with 8% of women in general. The study found that 20% had been told they were not at risk, while 1 in 50 had been refused a test. The following scenario examines the importance of inclusive health care and includes elements of communication, ethics and patient-centred care.

Scenario 2

Miss P presented for a new patient health check. She was a 30-year-old college lecturer, with no significant past or current medical history. The consultation included aspects of lifestyle to identify risk factors for coronary heart disease and cancer, including cervical cancer. When asked about her smear status, Miss P was open about her sexuality and stated she had not had a smear as her last nurse had told her she did not need one. Miss P was in a stable homosexual relationship and had never had sex with a man.

The nurse had experience of discussing sexual health with homosexual women so was comfortable in this consultation. She explained the importance of smears, their purpose, and the management of abnormal smears. The nurse gave Miss P all the relevant information to make an informed decision about the procedure, recording in the patient notes that Miss P had a low-risk — not a no-risk — of developing cervical cancer and that she had been advised to attend for a smear (NHS Cancer Screening Programme, 2008). Miss P attended for a smear as suggested. The nurse explained what she was doing at every stage of the procedure, including the receipt of the results. This first smear result showed signs of severe dyskariosis, which required further investigation. The nurse contacted Miss P and discussed the result. Miss P was very matter of fact about the result and attended all her clinic appointments and repeat smears at the surgery. She was grateful that the abnormality had been identified and encouraged her homosexual friends to also have smears tests.

In the scenario above a rushed appointment or lack of sensitivity or knowledge from the nurse could have resulted in Miss P leaving the surgery still under the impression that a smear was unnecessary. The severity of the abnormality could have resulted in invasive cancer if left untreated, requiring subsequent major surgery.

Anecdotally, homosexual women are often told they do not need a cervical smear test. This view is shared among the homosexual community as they may not have some of the risk factors for cervical cancer, such as being on the oral contraceptive pill (NHS Cancer Screening Programme, 2008). However it is still important to have a smear if they have other risk factors such as a high incidence of cigarette smoking (Stonewall, 2008). Some homosexual women may have had a heterosexual experience in the past, and some will be bisexual. Additionally, sharing sex aid toys is a risk for transmitting viral infections.

Nurses need to be sensitive to all patients and never make assumptions about their sexuality. Nurses must also be given sufficient time for appointments to allow patients to share any concerns and have questions answered, as has already been discussed in Chapter 1. The nurse who fails to follow national screening guidelines, resulting in a woman later developing invasive cancer, would be accountable for her actions (NMC, 2008).

Nurses have a responsibility to all their patients. It may be essential to stress to these patients that records are confidential, and to reassure patients that genitourinary medicine (GUM) clinic information is also confidential unless patients consent to sharing information with the GP.

The scenario below may not be relevant to all nurses as some practices might offer a full screening service. However in any consultation, ignorance about services is not an excuse for failing to deliver appropriate health advice.

Scenario 3

Mr J attended for travel advice. He was travelling to Thailand and required typhoid and hepatitis A vaccinations. The nurse gave Mr J the injections and information relating to travel health, supported by literature. Mr J rose to leave, and then stopped.

Mr J: 'Can I ask you something, nurse?'

Nurse: 'Yes, of course. What is it?'

Mr J: 'Can I be tested for HIV?'

Nurse [taken aback]: 'Sit down, and let's talk about this.'

Mr J explains that he is worried about HIV as he has never been tested. The nurse allows Mr J to finish his explanation.

Nurse: 'We can take the sample and send it to the lab, but it would be better for you to attend the sexual health clinic. They will offer you a full screen. This is confidential. They won't send us the results unless you consent, so there will

---

be nothing on your medical records. If you do have an infection, it is important that your past and present partners are also checked. We can't do that from the surgery.'

Mr J: 'Oh. Yes, I understand. Where will I have to go?'

The nurse provided Mr J with the relevant contact information, and ended the consultation.'

General health

There has been extensive research examining the health needs of homosexual men, yet this research is predominately concerned with their sexual behaviour and the prevention, treatment, and social policy implications of HIV and AIDS (Stonewall, 2009). Although homosexual and bisexual men have the same risks and concerns about their health as heterosexual men, they may not be comfortable talking about them.

This preoccupation with sexual health and HIV can have an impact on health service delivery to homosexual men. For example, a homosexual man might be celibate or in a monogamous relationship, yet his GP or nurse might continually give him information about safe sex because it is assumed that this is the individual's only health care need. The narrow focus on sexual activity can sometimes demonstrate to young men, or men who are discovering their sexuality, that being homosexual is just about sex. This can have an impact on relationships and on an overall sense of well being (Stonewall, 2009).

The majority of research concerned with other aspects of health care for homosexual men was mainly conducted in the early 1990s (Stonewall, 2009). It has been reported that homosexual men are concerned about issues relating to mental health, sexual behaviour and safety, weight issues and eating disorders, a lack of role models, and relationships. Some are also concerned about smoking, drinking, and drug and alcohol abuse (Stonewall, 2009).

Gay and bisexual men have the same risks and concerns about their health as heterosexual men, but may not be comfortable talking about them. One man surveyed stated: *'One of my biggest worries is that I would feel most uncomfortable talking with the GP about such things as testicular cancer etc or anything of a sexual nature because of the perceived (probably incorrect) stigma that might be attached as a consequence of my sexual orientation.'*

Nurses are in an ideal position during their consultations to introduce these topics. Well-men and new patient checks will usually include all aspects of general health and health promotion. Health promotion leaflets and resources can be accessed from the internet. Men can be directed to relevant websites if they wish to explore a topic in further depth. Websites that offer general health advice for gay men include Healthy Gay Life and Stonewall, which are excellent resources for information and support for men and women who are LGBT.

Ethnic minorities

Issues relating to ethnic minorities are discussed in Chapter 9.

Dealing with death

Homosexual, bisexual and transgender people who lose a partner through death or separation need the same bereavement counselling and support services as heterosexual men and women. The nurse should be empathetic and prioritise the consultation as noted in previous chapters.

Comments such as: '*We'd lived together for 22 years, and she was still referred to as "your friend" deny the close relationship between partners of the same sex.*' (Edwards, 2008). The consultation might involve a patient attending for a physical intervention, such as ear irrigation, but then evolve into bereavement counselling. In these instances it is important to understand the relationship dynamics in order to offer genuine support and empathy. The listening skills discussed in Chapter 2 are of paramount importance for this role.

Summary

Do not rush to the conclusion of heterosexuality. Use neutral language and allow patients to share their sexuality and concerns as they wish. The nurse should not aim to be able to identify or encourage a patient to disclose their sexuality, but to create an environment in which they will be comfortable to attend for help and support for all aspects of physical and/or mental health related to their sexuality. By indicating this level of openness and inclusiveness, practice nurses are in a prime position to create the safe environment required for good rapport and the disclosure of other significant information necessary for accurate diagnosis and treatment.

The following comment from the author's survey places sexuality in content:

'Finally I think it needs to be made clear that being gay is not a lifestyle choice - it's the way we are and I can't do anything about it without living a lie.'

Key points

- Do not rush to the conclusion of heterosexuality.
- Sexuality should not adversely affect patient care
- Respect patient confidentiality
- Be open and inclusive.

Asscheman H, Gooren LJ, Eklund PL (1989) Mortality and morbidity in transsexual patients with cross-gender hormone treatment. *Metabolism* **38**(9): 869–73

Edwards M (2008) *The Informed Practice Nurse* 2nd edn. Wiley, London

General Medical Council (2008) *Sexual orientation* www.gmc-uk.org/.../sexual-orientation.asp. accessed 1/4/2009

Neville S, Henrickson M (2006) Perceptions of lesbian, gay and bisexual people of primary healthcare services. *Journal of Advanced Nursing* **55**(4): 407–15

NHS Cancer Screening Programmes (2008) *NHS Cervical Screening programme*. www.cancerscreening.nhs.uk/cervical. accessed 25/1/2009

Nursing and Midwifery Council (2008) *The Code. Standards of conduct, performance and ethics for nurses and midwives*. NMC, London

Phillips-Angeles E, Wolfe P, Myers R et al (2004) Lesbian Health Matters: A Pap Test Education Campaign Nearly Thwarted by Discrimination. *Health Promotion Practice* **5**(3): 314–25

Royal College of Nursing & Unison (2004) *Not `just' a friend. Best practice guidance on health care for lesbian, gay and bisexual service users*. RCN & Unison, London

Steele LS, Tinmouth JM, Lu A (2006) Regular health care use by lesbians: a path analysis of predictive factors. *Family Practice* **23**(6): 631–6

Stonewall (2006a) *Women and general health needs*. Stonewall.org.uk

Stonewall (2006b) *How many lesbian, gay and bisexual people are there?* www.stonewall.org.uk/information_bank. accessed 4/9/2006

Stonewall & General Medical Council (2008) *Protecting patients. Your rights as lesbian, gay and bisexual people*. Stonewall & GMC, London

Stonewall (2008) *Women and cancer*. www.stonewall.org.uk accessed 16/7/2008

Stonewall (2009) *Men & general health needs*. www.stonewall.org.uk accessed 3/4/2009

Transgender Zone (2009) *Transgender View of Transgender People*. http://www. transgenderzone.com accessed 16/4/2009

Whittle S, Turner L, Alami M (2007) *Engendered Penalties: Transgender and Transsexual People's Experiences of Inequality and Discrimination*. Cabinet Office, London

Resources

Healthy Gay Life: *www.hgl.nhs.uk*

London Lesbian and Gay Switchboard: *020 7837 7324*

Stonewall: *www.stonewall.org.uk*

Queery: *www.queery.org.uk*

Transgender Zone: *www.transgenderzone.com*

CHAPTER 8

Delivering bad news

Bad news in relation to health can be described as any information that is likely to worsen a patient's view of their condition and may cause long lasting mental and behavioural problems. Bad news is a message that has the potential to shatter hopes and dreams, leading to a different lifestyle and future. Nurses are rarely taught how to deliver bad news. Although nurses do not usually deliver bad news relating to life threatening illnesses, for example such as cancer, there are occasions when they do deliver bad news for other reasons; this might be a diagnosis of diabetes, that a wound is infected with Methicillin Resistant *Staphylococcus Aureus* (MRSA) or a cervical smear result that requires further investigation. All of these examples can cause the patient anxiety.

When breaking bad news it is important to not make assumptions on behalf of patients (Hall, 2005). Everyone is different in their emotions, their reactions, and their perceptions of bad news; for example, for one patient hospital admission might be a relief, while for another it is bad news. Similarly, a diagnosis of diabetes could be a relief for one patient as it would explain their symptoms if they have been worried about a more sinister cause, while for another patient it may conjure up fears of amputation and blindness.

Personal aspects have an impact on how deeply nurses are able to care for their patients and how at ease they will be with the process of delivering bad news. The more often the nurse has to deal with this process, the more likely it is they will feel at ease in the situation. The following quotes are from oncology nurses and describe their feelings in relation to breaking bad news. Their feelings can relate and are relevant to practice nurses too (Tylee et al, 2009):

'It is easier once you have become a bit more practised at it.'

'I think one becomes quite skilled at it.'

'It's always painful and never easy.'

'It is an area that I tend to avoid.'

'*I am uncomfortable.*'

'*I don't really feel comfortable with bad news and I would rather someone else told them.*'

'*I feel inadequate and as though I don't have enough information.*'

'*I don't like to make people feel unhappy it is awful to have to do that.*'

Each nurse will have different coping mechanisms. Knowing the patient and having a good rapport can help.

Buckman's (1992) six-step guide is often used as a guide to breaking bad news (see *Box 8.1*). Some nurses become emotionally attached to certain patients or families. This can cause a dependency that is not beneficial to the patient or nurse, and can make supporting families in cases of bereavement a difficult experience for the nurse. The surviving family member/s might drift towards this nurse, resulting in consultations for a clinical reason being overshadowed by grief or anger.

How patients react

At the initial consultation the nurse may worry about what to say to the patient, how to say it, how to cope with the patient's reaction, how it is going to affect the nurse.

Box 8.1 Buckman's six-step guide to breaking bad news

S.P.I.K.E.S

Setting, listening skills
Patient's perception
Invite patient to share information
Knowledge transmission
Explore emotions and empathize
Summarize and strategize

Source: Buckman (1992)

Dealing with bad news is an essential skill for nurses where both verbal and non-verbal communication skills are important. Open body language, good eye contact and a welcoming expression can reassure anxious patients (Bryant, 2008). Use open questions to show interest and reflect back concerns to enable the patient to feel heard and feel valued. The nurse can support the patient and/or carer by establishing a rapport and recognising emotional distress and/or low mood (Towers, 2007). Key skills to manage a situation are listed in *Boxes 8.2* and *8.3*.

When bad news is delivered poorly the experience may stay in the patient's or family's mind long after the shock has been dealt with (McEnhill, 2008). Patients often feel denial and anger when they are given bad news. Delivering bad news also affects the news-giver. The nurse might be anxious about broaching or discussing a sensitive issue, but they can only do their best. It is easy to cause distress by giving bad news badly, and poor communication is the largest cause of complaints against medical and nursing staff (Lloyd-Williams and Lawrie, 2008).

Box 8.2 Key skills for dealing with bad news or sensitive issues

Good listening skills
Sympathetic body language
Knowledge to signpost
An ability to help but not get involved
Finding time

Source: Richards (2007), Towers (2007)

Box 8.3 Key listening skills

Focus on the other person
Keep still
Use appropriate body language
Give non-verbal response
Use questions
Summarise what you have heard
Use silence

Waiting

Patients are often anxious while waiting for results, for example blood results, X-rays or smears, especially if a previous result was abnormal. Some of the emotions patients might experience are listed in *Box 8.4*. The nurse should be aware of these in order to respond sensitively.

Box 8.4. Emotions patients might experience while awaiting results

Shock
Uncertainty
Fear
Anxiety
Hope
Depression

Denial

Delivering bad news at the patient's pace allows him the opportunity to block any further disclosure, hence the term 'denial'. It is generally a transient action and a way of coping with bad news. If bad news is given sensitively and at the recipient's pace, acceptance should follow (Breaking Bad News, 2008). Refer to Scenario 1.

Anger

Anger is a common reaction to bad news and is often linked to feelings of guilt and blame. This could be due to a diagnosis of terminal disease, a family member or friend who received poor care in hospital, or a sudden death. Nurses can be the recipients of a patient's anger from a previous event. The patient might be angry because a doctor has missed a diagnosis and offloads their anger on to the nurse. Although it is difficult and exhausting to listen to an angry torrent, listening can help dispel some of the emotion (Lloyd-Williams and Lawrie, 2008). The following steps are useful in handling anger:

• Acknowledge the anger (say what you see): '*I can see how angry you are about your husband's death*'

- Legitimise the anger if relevant: '*It must be hard for you that he went so quickly*'
- Find the true focus of the anger: '*I can see you are blaming the hospital, but can you explain why?*'
- Encourage expressions of feelings: '*Can you tell me how you are feeling just now?*'

Scenario 1

Mrs D was a 73-year-old smoker who was also a heavy drinker. She had a diagnosis of cancer of the tongue. She could not eat solid food, and found it painful to drink, so was managed with PEG feeds, supplemented with high calorie drinks. When she attended for a flu injection she asked ' ...how much worse will the pain get?' What could the nurse reply?

'Tell me about the pain' — describe whether the same, worse, constant.

'What painkillers do you take?' — check concordance and the need for stronger analgesia.

'What have the doctors said?' — assess her knowledge of the prognosis.

This is a difficult scenario as the prognosis is poor, The pain will get much worse and the analgesia is insufficient. The nurse was aware that Mrs D knew she had inoperable cancer and was aware there was no further treatment,but she still had hope — Mrs D was in denial of the palliative nature of the disease. This consultation resulted in the nurse listening to Mrs D, ascertaining her concerns, asking the doctor for improved pain relief and referral to the hospice service.

Grief

Grief can relate to facing loss of good health or restrictions on lifestyle associated with bad health, as well as bereavement. For example, a keen sportsman might grieve because he can no longer play football due to previous injury, or an elderly couple who were keen walkers but are now disabled with arthritis. In another example, a carer for a patient with dementia will grieve for the person they used to know.

The following scenario relates to a patient who has had an abnormal electrolyte result indicating chronic kidney disease (CKD), and will need a second test to confirm or exclude the condition. The patient is a known diabetic.

Scenario 2

Mr P attended a diabetic review accompanied by his wife.

Nurse: 'Hello Mr P, Mrs P. Please sit down, you look well today.'

Mr P: 'We've just come back from holiday.'

Nurse: 'You obviously had good weather. We need to have a chat about your blood results. How were you on the day of the test?' [Elicits whether or not Mr P was unwell on the day, which might affect the reading.]

Mr P: 'Same as always.'

Nurse: 'One of the tests suggests that your kidneys aren't working as well as they used to. In these cases we like to have a second blood test.'

Mr P: 'What does that mean?'

Nurse: 'We need to make sure the first test result is right. The body is like a car and parts wear out as we get older. We can discuss this when we have the next blood result.'

Mr P: 'And if that's bad, what happens then?'

Nurse: 'We'll go through that when we have the results. Would you like a leaflet to read?'

In the scenario above Mr P has been forewarned that he might have CKD so some of the grieving will already have taken place by the patient is reviewed (Bryant, 2008).

In other similar scenarios, the nurse can help by taking an empathetic approach and encouraging the patient to talk through his concerns. For example by asking the patient: *'I can see that you are having difficulty in coming to terms with the changes in your life. Would it help to talk?'* (Breaking Bad News 2008).

Consider scenario 3 where the nurses who undertook consultations with the bereaved had to manage anger, grief and blame. It would be reasonable to offer such patients an early appointment to be a listening ear if no

Scenario 3

Mr J was a 60-year-old man who suffered from asthma, hypertension and sleep apnoea. He was concordant with all his therapies and attended all reviews. A home visit was requested early on Monday morning as Mr J had abdominal pain. Half an hour later the visit was cancelled as his wife had called an ambulance. Mr J died that afternoon following a ruptured aortic aneurysm.

Consider the emotions of Mrs J and his son Tim, aged 26. Both were angry at Mr J for leaving them so suddenly. Tim had anger and guilt that he was not at the bedside when his father died. Mrs J felt guilt and blame that she had not called the ambulance in the early hours of the morning.

Mrs J attended for her smear test two months after Mr J died. She was tearful and still angry.

To manage this scenario would you:

- Perform the smear test and block out the emotion?
- Defer the smear and listen to the patient?
- Do the smear and refer the patient to a counsellor?
- Defer the smear, listen and refer?
- Not know what to do?

counselling service is available. This might avoid a later need for referral to the mental health service. Any screening or chronic disease review can be deferred until the patient feels stable. The nurse must respond to each patient as an individual as each has a different need.

Handling a difficult consultation

The nurse must be prepared when a patient is due for a consultation and bad news is due to be given. It is essential to:
- Confirm the medical facts of the case: for example, post operative laparotomy for bowel cancer
- Ensure that all necessary information is available: for example, wound swab results
- Try to create an environment in which the patient is comfortable: for example, a quiet room with no interruptions
- Ensure privacy and openness: as above, but also have a box of tissues to offer if necessary

There are several factors that can affect the consultation before it even begins (Bryant, 2008). The nurse who has a busy surgery may overlook these factors. Always consider the patient:

- How has their day been so far and how do they feel?
- Are there family or work problems?
- How long has the patient been waiting for his/her appointment?
- How long has the patient been waiting in the waiting room?
- Have there been any difficulties getting test results?

The nurse carrying out the consultation may have her/his own issues, for example if they have just seen a difficult patient, or if there is a backlog of patients, or if the nurse is simply having a bad day. The above issues can disrupt even the best-planned consultation.

In order to achieve understanding and manage a difficult consultation where you will be breaking bad news to a patient, consider the following (Bryant, 2008; gp-training.net 2009):

- Speak clearly, using non-medical terminology
- Write down any technical terms if necessary
- Find out the patient's views and health beliefs
- Assess the patient's understanding of their medical condition, the possible outcome of an assessment, prognosis and other options
- Discuss future strategies.

It has been reported that typically about 50% of patients or relatives do not understand information they are given concerning diagnosis, cause and likely outcome of their condition (Ley, 1982 cited by Bryant 2008). If the patient asks you questions you do not know the answer to, do not be afraid to admit you do not have all the knowledge. Say '*I'm sorry*' or '*I don't know*'.

Pacing and shared control:

- Get to the point and do not waffle
- Allow for pauses — silences are useful. Listen to the patient and watch out for non-verbal cues
- Give the patient time to absorb the information
- Let the patient take some of the lead and involve them in management decisions
- Allow the patient to ask questions.

Responding to emotions:

- Touch the patient/relative only if appropriate
- Reassure that it is alright to cry — have the tissues on the desk
- Use eye contact and non-verbal communication
- Show your own emotion — you can cry too, but within limits. Remember it is their grief and not yours
- Offer continuing support and practical advice. This could include referral to support groups.

Closure:

- Summarise at the end of the discussion
- Finish with positive points
- Close discussion by inviting questions
- Document what has been discussed.

Box 8.5 lists some tips on breaking bad news, which supports the above guidance. The following scenario places this list in perspective.

Scenario 4

Mrs B attended for a new patient health check. She had no relevant medical history but her body mass index (BMI) was noted to be 35.47, with a waist measurement of 102 cm. Practice policy was to offer a fasting blood sugar (FBS) test to all patients with a BMI greater than 30. The blood result showed a FBS of 6.9. A repeat FBS test was 7.1. Mrs B was referred to the practice nurse for management.

The nurse had the blood results to hand (1) and allocated a 30-minute appointment for this first visit (2). Mr B accompanied his wife (4). Mrs B suspected she could have diabetes, as her sister had been diagnosed two years before (5). The nurse explained the diagnosis, supported with literature to ensure Mrs and Mr B understood what had been said (9).

At this first visit limited information was given, with further appointments booked to continue the education (B). Mrs B was informed that there is no such thing as mild diabetes and it was important to reduce the blood sugars (D, G).

Box 8.5. How to break bad news

Do:

1. Have the facts to hand
2. Clear enough time
3. Control potential interruptions. Block telephone calls, use 'do not disturb' signs, or ask colleagues not to interrupt
4. Check if the patient wishes anyone else be present
5. Clarify what the patient already knows
6. Be prepared to follow the patient's agenda
7. Observe and acknowledge the patient's emotional reactions,
8. Stop if the patient indicates they do not wish to continue
9. Check the patient understands what has been said
10. Listen
11. Use open questions

Do not:
A. Make assumptions about the impact of the news, the patient's readiness to hear news, priorities, and understanding
B. Give too much information at one time
C. Decide what is most important for the patient
D. Give inappropriate reassurance
E. Answer questions unless the facts are to hand
F. Hurry the consultation
G. Use euphemisms, for example 'mild diabetes'
H. Block emotional expression from the patient
I. Break the news to relatives without telling the patient
J. Agree to relatives' demands that information is withheld from the patient

Source: Breaking Bad News (2008)

In scenario 4 Mrs B was still shocked by the diagnosis, even though she expected it. The word diabetes may conjure images of amputations and blindness, and is thus very bad news for some patients. Practice nurses are the people who usually break this news to the patient, and need the skills to manage this sensitively. The patient needs time to come to terms with a diagnosis that will affect their lifestyle for a lifetime. It is important to resist the temptation to fill a silence with more information, as little information will be retained on this occasion. Patients understand and retain information better if given in small manageable amounts, and are aware of its importance (Bryant, 2008).

Nurses manage and support patients with a variety of prolonged and chronic disease including cancer, diabetes, chronic obstructive pulmonary disease, asthma and coronary heart disease. These patients may have a succession of bad news, with the associated continuing fear/anxiety. Family and carers may also need support during this time. A good relationship between the patient, significant others and the nurse is crucial. Rabow and McPhee (2000) reinforce the need to coordinate the disease with personal goals. Consider scenario 5.

Blocking behaviour and managing difficult questions

Blocking behaviour relates to the nurse using tactics to prevent discussion of the bad news. These include:

* Offering advice and reassurance before the main problem has been identified
* Explaining to the patient that feeling distress is normal
* Considering the physical, but not the psychological, aspects
* Changing the topic.

Scenario 5

Pat had been attending the surgery two to three times a week for dressing of a postoperative laparotomy wound for some months. The wound had reopened following surgery for colon cancer and chemotherapy was being delayed. The wound was now approximately 15 cm x 10 cm. During the preceding consultations the nurses had explored Pat's feelings about her diagnosis and were aware that she knew that further treatment was unlikely.

Nurse: 'How are you feeling today?'

Pat: 'I'd really like to go away for a break.' [looks sad]

Nurse: 'What's stopping you doing this?' [allows patient to elaborate and share her concerns]

Pat: 'I can't go away, with this wound. The dressing won't last a week.'

Nurse: 'That's not a problem. We can arrange for you to see the local nurse as a temporary patient if you let us know where you're going.' [coordinates disease with personal goals]

Pat: 'Can you?' [face lights up]

Nurse: 'Discuss it with your husband, and let us know where you're going.'

Pat's husband booked a week in a cottage where they could take their dog. He found the contact number for the local surgery and arranged for Pat to be seen by their practice nurses. Her own nurses arranged a supply of dressings to accompany a letter explaining the wound management. This arrangement worked well, and Pat had several further short breaks. Her psychological health improved, which may have impacted upon her wound healing. The wound healed and her quality of life dramatically improved.

There are some questions that the nurse does not wish to be asked, the main one being: *'Am I dying?'*. Nurses can be asked any question at any time and need to be prepared to respond. Consider scenario 6.

Barriers to an effective consultation

There can always be barriers during a consultation. Specific ones relating to delivering or sharing bad news include (Towers, 2007):

- Avoid using a relative or friend to interpret for a patient whose first language is not English, both because of confidentiality and because they might misinterpret what has been said (see Chapter 9)
- The nurses themselves might be afraid of opening emotions difficult to handle and be unable to cope emotionally with the outcome
- Blocking ignores the signs that the patient wishes to talk
- Changing the subject also blocks the issue
- Selectively focusing on a physical issue, such as pain relief, to avoid the psychological problems
- Referring the patient to a doctor for support
- Offering false reassurances
- Trivialising, making the patient's concerns seem insignificant
- Asking closed questions, which prevents the patient opening up and maintains control of the conversation.

Scenario 6

Julie's husband had a diagnosis of bowel cancer. He was in hospital having deteriorated and an MRI scan had been taken. A few days later Julie attended for her diabetic check with the nurse. Julie did not know what was happening, so asked the nurse to phone the ward. She was informed that the cancer had spread to the brain. The nurse was unable to repeat the ward information but her body language suggested bad news. Julie asked: 'Has the cancer spread?' When the nurse said 'Yes' Julie screamed and started crying.

Why did it happen?
There was a good rapport between Julie and the nurse. The nurse was uncomfortable making enquiries on Julie's behalf, but understood her concerns. Neither the nurse nor Julie were expecting bad news.

What action was taken?
The nurse sat with Julie and allowed her to share her feelings. They cried together. Julie left the room knowing she could discuss this with the nurse at any time.

Implications
Should the ward have given the nurse the bad news? Could the nurse have pretended she did not know the answer? In this instance Julie was prepared for the news when she visited her husband later than day.

Reflection
Although this was a difficult situation, the nurse acted in Julie's best interests. However, there is the issue of confidentiality, as the husband might have wished to keep this news from Julie. However Julie asked a question, and the nurse answered it honestly. Patients often use euphemisms such as: 'I won't be bothering you for long' when they think they are dying. This type of hint allows the nurse to sensitively explore the patient's feelings and concerns.

Summary

There is no right or wrong way to broach a sensitive issue but a considered approach will help ensure the patient can move forward (Richards, 2007). Ask the patient to repeat or paraphrase what has been said to ensure they understand the implications of the bad news. Although delivering bad news is often difficult it is a skill that can be developed and can improve with experience.

Key points

- Plan how to deliver the news
- What does the patient already know?
- Good listening is essential
- The nurse does not need to answer 'why me?'

Breaking Bad News (2008) *Breaking Bad News*. www.breakingbadnews.co.uk accessed 13/12/2008

Bryant L (2008) Breaking bad news. *Practice Nurse* **35**(5): 3 37–42

Buckman, R (1992) *How to Break Bad News A guide for Health Care Professionals*. Johns Hopkins University Press, Baltimore

gp-training.net (2009) *Breaking bad news*. www.gp-training.net/...badnews.htm accessed 22/2/2009

Hall A (2005) Breaking bad news. *Journal of Community Nursing* **19**(9): 30–1

Lloyd-Williams M, Lawrie I (2008) Breaking bad news to patients and relatives. *BMJ Learning*. www.learning.bmj.com. accessed 11/10/2008

McEnhill LS (2008) Breaking bad news of cancer to people with learning disabilities. *British Journal of Learning Disabilities* **36:** 157–64

Rabow MW, McPhee SJ (2000) *Beyond breaking bad news: Helping patients who suffer*. http://student.bmj.com/back_issues/0300/education/65.html

Richards S (2007) How to address sensitive issues. *Practice Nurse* **33**(2): 31–3

Towers R (2007) Providing psychological support for patients with cancer. *Nursing Standard* **22**(12): 50–7

Tylee J, McKeown S, Tylee P (2009) *Registered Nurses' Experiences of Breaking Bad News: A Phenomenological Study*. http://www.education4skills.com/jtylee/breaking_bad_news.html

CHAPTER 9

Cultural diversity

The United Kingdom is a multicultural society that includes many ethnic groups as well as gypsies and travellers, refugees and asylum seekers. Practice populations across the nation will vary dramatically. Some may have a high ethnic population from one country, some a wide variation, and others a high proportion of asylum seekers. Regardless of ethnicity, all patients are entitled to equity in health care.

Nurses need to understand the ethnicity of their practice population to be able to engage their patients during a consultation. This includes understanding the specific health problems of certain groups and their underlying health beliefs (Dhami and Sheikh, 2008). This chapter offers guidance on consultation skills where ethnicity and culture may be a challenge within the practice.

Race relations legislation

Race relations legislation makes both direct and indirect discrimination illegal on the grounds of:

• Race
• Colour
• Nationality
• Ethnic origin

(General Medical Council, 2008)

Good communication, both verbal and non-verbal, is the cornerstone of high quality, patient-centred care (Dhami & Sheikh, 2009). The importance of body language is discussed in Chapter 2. Even patients with poor spoken English skills will detect negative posture or facial expressions. Conversely, a welcoming smile is understood by anyone, irrespective of language (see Chapter 1).

Patient's perspective

'When I am asked where I come from, I always say I am a Greek Cypriot born in England. I cannot deny this, and if people feel the need to ask this question, it is obvious that I must either look different or behave differently or else they wouldn't have asked. But I am proud to be a Greek Cypriot.'

(Papadopoulos, 2000).

This quote highlights the importance of treating each person as an individual. Asking about background can be a useful way to develop the nurse/patient rapport. It is also important to use positive body language to show genuine interest in the person and their culture.

Body language and non-verbal communication

It is helpful to have an idea of how different cultures use differing non-verbal communication. The following examples are accessed from Management Sciences for Health (2009a).

Facial expressions

Some Chinese people may smile when discussing something sad or uncomfortable. It is therefore important to observe tone of voice and other body language during the consultation.

Head gestures

In Lebanon the signal for 'yes' may be a nod of the head, while 'no' can be a sharp point upward with raised eyebrows. Saudis may signal 'yes' by swivelling their head from side to side, and 'no' by tipping their head back and clicking their tongue. It is therefore essential to clarify whether the patient is saying 'Yes' or 'No'.

Hand and arm gestures

The circular 'OK' sign made with fingers is interpreted as money in Japan, as it is the shape of a coin. However in other countries around the world, including some Eastern European ones, this gesture indicates a bodily orifice and is highly offensive. The sign means 'zero' or 'nothing' in some European countries, Argentina and Zimbabwe. Be careful using the thumbs up sign for 'OK', as although it might be suitable for some cultures, it has a vulgar meaning to Iranians.

Touching

In the Middle East and some African cultures, it is the custom to use the left hand for bodily hygiene. Never offer the left hand to shake hands.

Eye contact

Although eye contact is considered a valuable non-verbal communication skill, Robertson (2008) reminds us that in some cultures eye contact would be considered disrespectful. However, in other cultures, refusing to make eye contact is a sign of disrespect. Take the lead from the patient.

Use arm gestures with caution and be careful interpreting facial expressions. Do not force a patient to make eye contact as this might suggest he is being disrespectful. Nurses who work with different ethnic groups and cultures may already be aware of cultural differences. Those who are new in an area might find it helpful to investigate local cultures.

Cultural issues - consent

Regard must be given to the cultural backgrounds within the practice population when considering informed consent for both adults and children. Difficulties with language can clearly have an impact when obtaining consent for treatment.
For example:
* Explaining and obtaining consent for any physical examination, including cervical smears
* Administering vaccinations, both for child and adult immunisations
* Devising a management plan for any chronic disease, especially where medication can be altered, such as insulin or in acute asthma
* Providing travel advice, including the choice of malaria prophylaxis.

An interpreter may be required for patients whose first language is not English. This may be a child or relative, which creates problems with respect to sensitive issues and patient confidentiality, although without an interpreter, the patient is unable to give informed consent. This is discussed in detail overleaf.

Interpreters

Language is often a major barrier to accessing high quality health care. Interpreters can be used face-to-face or via the telephone through services such as Language Line (discussed below). According to Dhami and Sheikh (2008), these services will help reduce tensions and should enhance the patients' experience of care. However, it is difficult for a person at the other end of a phone to assess body language.

A study of district nurses found resistance towards using formal resources, including interpreters and Language Line, with staff having a lack of confidence in these services and concerns about confidentiality (Peckover and Chidlaw, 2007). However the study reported that district nurses who receive training to work with interpreters are more confident and make use of the services more frequently. This is also pertinent for allied nurses. Nurses who work with ethnic minorities should make an effort to access training as this could improve consultation skills enormously.

A Department of Health (DH)(2008) study noted that patients need to be informed about the role of the interpreter, need to have confidence in the interpreter and the advice they receive.

Face-to-face interpreters can be beneficial but they may need to be booked in advance which may not be possible for an emergency appointment. In these instances, the use of an informal interpreter may be necessary. The patient will require a longer appointment to allow for translation, especially if a telephone service is used.

Language Line

Language Line is an interpretation service operated over the telephone, where an interpreter listens to the limited English speaking patient (LEP), analyses the message and accurately conveys its original meaning to the nurse.

Professionally trained and tested Language Line Services interpreters do not interpret word-for-word, but meaning-for-meaning, which means that non-English conversations can seem to take longer. Many English concepts that are communicated in one or two words can take several phrases to accurately describe in another language, and vice versa. Telephone interpreting offers a fast response when urgent or unexpected language barriers crop up.

To access this service, the practice or clinic must be registered with Language Line (see Resources). When the nurse consults with the LEP in a face-to-face situation she will:

- Dial the Language Line Services designated toll-free number
- Request the language the patient speaks through an easy-to-use interactive voice response (IVR) system
- Use the Language Line Phone, speakerphone, or pass her handset back and forth when the interpreter is connected.
  Box 9.1 offers guidelines for working with interpreter.

Scenario 1

Mr and Mrs A recently joined the practice. They are asylum seekers from Somalia. Neither has a good command of the English language, and none of the staff spoke their dialect. The practice has a large population of ethnic minority patients, and is registered with Language Line.

The couple attended for a new patient health check with the nurse. The nurse welcomed them with a smile and gestured for them to be seated. They were unable to complete a health questionnaire but Mrs A was evidently pregnant. The nurse was unable to obtain past and current medical histories, although she managed to communicate that she wished to weigh and measure them, and check their blood pressure. It was important to refer Mrs A to the midwifery service, so the nurse telephoned the free phone number and was put in contact with the appropriate interpreter. The interpreter managed to elicit the relevant medical information about both patients, including Mrs A's expected date of delivery. The nurse then referred Mrs A to the community midwife for ongoing care. Mr A was experiencing mental health problems that required medical intervention, and was referred to the GP.

No personal interpreter was available, so the appointment was extended to allow for the telephone interpretation service. The nurse used non-verbal communication to welcome the couple and undertake the simple measurements. She would not, however, be able to gain information about health status, current medication and presenting complaints without an interpreter.

Face-to-face interpreters

Professional interpreters are trained to convey messages without distortion from their own beliefs and prejudices. An on-site interpretation service is a more appropriate solution for a consultation that is pre-planned and needs face-to-face interaction. A professional interpreter service should:
- Be accessible and comprehensive
- Offer reliable and professional highly qualified and experienced interpreters

- Be culturally sensitive to the gender and dialect of the patient
- Be confidential and secure
- Offer a personal approach that can be particularly beneficial in highly sensitive situations
- Be able to use non-verbal and visual communication to help with complex and detailed issues

Face-to-face interpretation allows the nurse to assess the patient's body language, especially facial expressions and hand gestures. For example, the patient is able to point to a specific area of pain.

Reliance on family members is not recommended, especially for sensitive issues such as sexual health or contraception (Dhami and Sheikh, 2008). A professional interpreter has additional skills and training that family members may not have. Avoid using a relative or friend to interpret for a patient whose first language is not English due to concerns about confidentiality and because they might misinterpret what has been said. Children should never be used as interpreters because of the risk of mistakes

---

Box 9.1 Guidelines for working with interpreters

- Hold a brief pre-interview meeting with the interpreter. Agree where the interpreter will sit and explain the background to the consultation, for example starting the patient on warfarin.
- Establish a good working relationship with the interpreter. If possible try to use the same interpreter although this may be difficult in practice.
- Allow enough time for the consultation. What may take a few words to explain in one language may require longer paraphrasing in another.
- Do not say anything that the patient should not hear, but expect the interpreter to interpret everything that the nurse, patient and family member will say.
- Speak clearly in a normal voice at a steady pace.
- Watch the patient's body language when they answer a question; do not watch the interpreter.
- Avoid jargon and technical terms. The interpreter might understand what is meant, but have difficulty in the translation.
- Ask only one question at a time to prevent confusing the patient.
- Be prepared to repeat the question if the answer suggests the question was misinterpreted.

(Management Sciences for Health 2009b)

---

in translation (Dhami and Sheikh, 2009). However some patients may feel more comfortable having a family member present during the consultation, and this may be a child (Suresh and Suresh, 2008).

A DH report noted that bilingual children from minority ethnic groups were found to act as informal interpreters between the GP and parents when their parents have little or no fluency in English (Cohen, 2007). Interpretation on behalf of parents, siblings and in relation to their own health can also occur during nursing consultations, with the associated concerns about misdiagnosis or miscommunication. Cohen (2007) also reported that where there was a linguistic concern, there was preference for a trained Health Advocate to attend and mediate the consultation.

Untrained interpreters may not convey the correct information from patient to nurse/nurse to patient. It is worth remembering that although some health promotion materials are available in different languages, people may not be able to read in their known first language.

The consultation

A government report investigating primary care experiences of black and ethnic minority (BEM) people identified that BEM patients are less likely than the general population to feel that they had sufficient time with their GP (DH, 2008). This feeling can be transferable to nursing consultations. Poor communication can impact on the length of consultation time needed. Consideration of length of appointments was discussed in Chapter 1. Just because some BEM patients have lower expectations of nurses (DH, 2008) does not mean that the nurse has to meet these expectations. This is an opportunity to redress these expectations and deliver high quality care.

One issue with BEM patients is that some may not always regard appointment times as rigid and may arrive late for appointments. Should they be turned away or 'fitted in'? If turned away, a child may miss an important immunisation. However, if seen, it may either:

(a) set a precedent and they will always come when they feel like it, or
(b) send the message to other patients that they can also come at any time.

The practice should try to devise a policy to deal with these situations that prevents the nurse being placed in an uncomfortable position.

The nurse might be presented with a patient with limited spoken English, requiring an emergency electrocardiogram (ECG), with only a family member as interpreter. Scenario 2 highlights the value of having a family member present during a consultation.

Scenario 2

Mr S presented to the doctor with chest pain. The doctor then referred him to the nurse for an ECG. The nurse ushered Mr S and his son into the consulting room where the ECG machine was already prepared. She explained the procedure while his son translated. Mr S understood that he had to remove his upper clothes and lie on the bed. The nurse demonstrated that she would be putting sticky pads on his limbs and chest, and proceeded with the ECG. On completion Mr S redressed and the nurse explained that the doctor wished to see the result. This was translated and both men were directed to a waiting area.

In this situation time was at a premium and a family member was an appropriate interpreter. This was particularly relevant as Mr S was admitted to hospital for cardiac assessment

Health beliefs

People have their own health beliefs and practices based on cultural background. For instance, some Muslims might not accept health promotion because they do not believe they can stop something happening if God has preordained it for them, while others will follow the Prophet Mohammed's guidance to maintain their health (Odeh, 2008). The nurse must gauge each person's beliefs and accept his or her decisions.

The DH (2008) study reported that it was often difficult to get BEM patients involved in traditional preventative health and self management programmes. There are however projects in inner city areas that successfully address this issue (DH 2008). Nurses can liaise with community health educators and link workers to improve patients' self-care. The development of a broader understanding around inequalities, human and citizenship rights, while also promoting the development of skills, is needed to bring about change at the patient/client level (Papadopoulos et al 1998, cited by Berjon-Aparicio, 2007).

Practice nurses may find it difficult to discuss sexual health matters with Orthodox Jewish women as they may be perceived as taboo topics (Berjon-Aparicio, 2007). It is impossible for nurses to know all about every different cultural group or even all about one specific cultural group but training in transcultural issues will help.

The health beliefs of a Jehovah's Witness are linked to religion and include practising a healthy lifestyle (see Box 9.2). This knowledge can

---

Box 9.2 Health beliefs of a Jehovah's Witness

No smoking
No overindulgence of food or alcohol
No sex before marriage
No blood products, neither that eaten nor tranfused

(Fowles 2008)

---

help guide a consultation, as it is relevant when prescribing medication or dressings and discussing lifestyle issues. In respect of illness and/or dying, followers are comforted by their religion. Do not be afraid to ask them about their feelings as they are guided by the bible.

Goal setting

Realistic goal setting can aid patient concordance to a management plan. This is particularly relevant when discussing dietary modifications with some patients. It is important to be aware of cultural and religious norms and try to adapt advice accordingly, as shown in the following scenario.

Scenario 3

Mrs K had a body mass index of 35, which is categorised as obese, and was recently diagnosed with type 2 diabetes. She saw the diabetes trained nurse who ascertained the reason for the consultation, which was to discuss dietary and lifestyle issues.

Nurse: 'Hello Mrs K. Let's start at the beginning and look at what you usually eat and drink.'

Mrs K lived with her husband in his family house. She liked sweet carbonated drinks and had sugar in her tea. Although the family were vegetarian, her mother-in- law cooked with ghee, a type of clarified butter. There had been several family weddings over the previous 3 months and Mrs K admitted she probably ate more than she would normally.

The nurse discussed healthy eating guidelines.

Nurse: 'How do think you could improve your diet?'

Mrs K: 'I could have less sugar I suppose.'

Nurse: 'How can you do this?'

Mr K: 'Perhaps stop sugary drinks?

Nurse: 'That would be a good idea. And what about changing from ghee to oil?

Mrs K: Oh. I don't think my mother-in-law would like that. She does all the cooking.

In this instance the nurse must respect the family culture and offer Mrs K the appropriate advice and support to reduce her weight and blood sugars, allowing her to identify possible changes. Delivering a structured education programme to hard to reach BEM groups is a challenge for all health professionals.

Alternative treatments

Some cultures prefer herbal or traditional remedies to Western medicines. For example 50% of African-Caribbean participants in one study were reported to believe that alternative remedies were more effective cures for their hypertension than Western medicines (Higginbottom and Mathers 2006, cited by Higginbottom, 2008). Some rejected Western medicines completely, while others took a combination of self-prescribed herbal and prescribed Western medicines.

This has implications for all prescribed medications. The nurse has the opportunity to discuss treatment concordance with the patient at every consultation. If the nurse does not ask about alternative treatment, the patient might not volunteer this information. As the chemical constituents of many herbal remedies are unknown, it might be necessary to find safer alternatives to some drugs.

Chaperones

See Chapter 3 for general and specific issues relating to chaperones.

Deaf and hard of hearing

There are approximately 100 000 deaf people in the UK belonging to ethnic minority groups without fluent English (Freeney et al 1999). This population is doubly isolated by their hearing loss and barriers created by language, culture, religion and racism. See Chapter 6 for tips on communicating with deaf people.

Learning disabilities

It is important to remember to include people with learning disabilities when considering minority groups. Refer to Chapter 6 for consultation skills for patients with a learning disability.

Sexual orientation

Lesbian bisexual gay and transexual (LBGT) members of minority ethnic groups might be less well served than the general population. Nurses will encounter family members who find it hard coming to terms with their son, daughter, sister or brother's sexuality. An appropriately edited version of 'A Guide for Families and Friends of Lesbians and Gays' can help nurses to support this group; the guide is now available in booklet form in Urdu as well as an audiocassette version in Hindi (see FFLAG in resources). See Chapter 7 for general information relating to sexual orientation.

Domestic violence services are mainly targeted to meet the needs of BEM heterosexual women but a study conducted in London reported that BEM LBGT people were more likely to experience physical abuse, more likely to experience harassment from a stranger and were equally likely to have experienced verbal abuse compared to their white LBGT counterparts (Fish, 2007). Nurses need to be alert to the physical and psychological signs of domestic violence and not be afraid to raise the topic.

Gypsies and travellers

Small scale localised studies suggest that gypsy travellers (also known as gypsies, travellers, Romanies or the Roma people) have poorer health status than non-travellers but reliable evidence on the health of adults is sparse (Parry et al, 2004). Travellers' health beliefs and attitudes to health services demonstrate a cultural pride in self-reliance. Parry et al (2004) found widespread communication difficulties between health workers and gypsy travellers, with defensive expectation of racism and prejudice. However positive experiences of health professionals who were perceived to be culturally well informed and sympathetic were highly valued. It is important that nurses who work with these communities have an understanding of their culture and appropriate ways to act and communicate.

Most women from gypsy and travelling communities would prefer to see a female health professional for an appointment. Most practice nurses are female, which can encourage women to access smears or family planning advice. This is an excellent opportunity to promote both their own and the family's health. Consider scenario 4.

Scenario 4

Mrs S was a 54-year-old woman who registered with the practice after moving to a council run travellers' site. She had not completed a health questionnaire so the nurse explained the rationale for asking about past and present medical history. Having recorded the relevant data the nurse expanded the consultation.

Nurse: 'When was your last smear?'

Mrs S: 'I don't believe in them.'

Nurse: 'Is there a particular reason for this?'

Mrs S: 'What will be will be. I don't want anybody messing with me.'

Nurse: 'It is an important test. It can be a little uncomfortable, but only for a few minutes. Any of the nurses can do this for you. Think about it. You can come back and talk about it if you have any questions.'

The nurse allowed Mrs S to consider having a smear, but did not try to coerce her. She noted on the records that Mrs S had been advised to have a smear and would reinforce this during future consultations (see Chapter 3).

Missing appointments

Gypsies and travellers may miss appointments due to poor literacy and/ or cultural differences. For example, gypsies and travellers may not use calendars or diaries, and lifestyles may not be based around the usual 9.00am to 5.00pm timings. Consider alternatives to written communication. It may be better to remind these patients about any appointments they have by phone or face-to-face.

Asylum seekers and refugees

A refugee is an asylum seeker whose application for asylum has been granted by the Home Office. Both refugee and asylum seekers are often psychologically and physically traumatised. They need empathy and sensitivity during consultations. All the issues relating to interpreters discussed above are relevant here.

Information giving to all groups

Jackson and Skinner (2007) studied the outcome of Somali patients having audio information recorded in their own language by the interpreter onto a digital recording device (DRD) following a consultation. The DRDs were useful for remembering advice given, reinforcing instructions on medication and appointment times, especially for older people. This method is worth exploring for practices with a high ethnic population who use interpreters.

Health service information is now routinely translated into ethnic minority languages and in a similar way, materials should be provided for a population that is recognised as having poor levels of literacy. Audiotapes or audio CDs could be more appropriate than printed information. Detailed oral explanation of how to take any prescribed medication is essential as many adults cannot read the printed instructions.

Summary

Never make assumptions about an individual's ability to understand on the basis of their colour or dress. Second level migrants may be impossible to distinguish from new ones (Dhami and Sheikh, 2009). Patient-held records could improve continuity of care with transient gypsies and travellers. This is especially relevant for child health records and chronic disease management. Utilise professional interpreters where possible but family members might be the most convenient on occasion. However, beware of misconstruction of information. Respect each person's culture.

Key points

* Consider the wide range of cultural diversity in the practice population
* Understand and respect each culture
* Use a professional interpreting service where possible.

Berjon-Aparicio S (2007) Cervical screening in an Orthodox Jewish community

Nursing Standard **21**(28): 44-9

Cohen S (2007) MCH 20-07: *Primary Health Care Services for Children from Ethnic Minority Groups*. London, DH

Department of Health (2008) *No Patient Left Behind: how can we ensure world class primary care for black and minority ethnic people?* London, DH

Dhami S & Sheikh A (2008) Health promotion: reaching ethnic minorities. *Practice Nurse* **36**(8): 21-5

Dhami S & Sheikh A (2009) Ethnicity and access to healthcare. *Practice Nurse* **37**(1): 40-4

Fish J (2007) *Reducing health inequalities for lesbian, gay, bisexual and trans people - briefings for health and social care staff*. London, DH

Fowles G (2008) *Basic beliefs of Jehovah's Witnesses*. www.watchtower.org accessed 17/4/2009

Freeney M, Cook R, Hale B et al. (1999) *Working in partnership to implement section 21 of the Disability Discrimination Act 1995 across the National Health Service*. London, Department of Health

General Medical Council (2008) *Race equality issues*. www.gmc-uk.org/...race_equality_ issues accessed 8/1/2009

Higgingbottom G (2008) "I didn't tell them. Well, they never ask". Lay understandings of hypertension and their impact on chronic disease management: implications for nursing practice in primary care. *Journal of Research in Nursing* **13**(2): 89-99

Jackson M & Skinner J (2007) Improving consultations in general practice for Somali patients: a qualitative study. *Diversity in Health and Social Care* **4**(1): 61-7

Management Sciences for Health (2009a) *Non-verbal communication*. http://erc.msh.org accessed 25/3/2009

Management Sciences for Health (2009b) *Working with an interpreter*. http://erc.msh.org accessed 25/3/2009

Odeh Y (2008) Arab Muslims' Health Beliefs and Practices. *Journal of Transcultural Nursing* **19**(3): 284-91

Papadopoulos I (2000) An Exploration of Health Beliefs, Lifestyle Behaviours, and Health

Needs of the London-Based Greek Cypriot Community. *Journal of Transcultural Nursing* **11**(3): 182-90

Parry G, Van Cleemput P, Peters J et al (2004) *The Health Status of Gypsies & Travellers in England*. Summary of a report to the Department of Health. University of Sheffield

Peckover S & Chidlaw RG (2007) The (un)-certainties of district nurses in the context of cultural diversity. *Journal of Advanced Nursing* **58**(4): 377-85

Robertson K (2008) *The importance of communication skills*. Practice nurse CPD. BMJ Learning. http://learning.bmj.com accessed 20/10/08

Suresh K & Suresh R (2008) *Tips on one-to-one interactions*. BMJ Learning. Practice Nurse CPD. www.learning.bmj.com accessed 21/10/2008

Resources

Asthma UK www.asthma.org.uk

Interpreter service (via Language Line) for callers to Adviceline

08457 010203

British Heart Foundation www.bhf.org.uk

Diabetes UK www.diabetes.org.uk

Information materials in English and 9 other languages

FFLAG www.fflag.org.uk

Language Line www.languageline.co.uk

Commission for Racial Equality

Manchester:Arndale House, The Arndale Centre, Manchester, M4 3AQ

T: 0161 829 8100 (non helpline calls only) F: 0161 829 8110

info@equalityhumanrights.com

London:3 More London, Riverside Tooley Street, London, SE1 2RG

T: 020 3117 0235 (non helpline calls only) F:0207 407 7557

info@equalityhumanrights.com

Cardiff: 3rd floor, 3 Callaghan Square, Cardiff, CF10 5BT

T: 02920 447710 (non helpline calls only) Textphone 029 20447713

F: 02920 447712 wales@equalityhumanrights.com

Glasgow: The Optima Building, 58 Robertson Street, Glasgow, G2

8DU T:0141 228 5910 (non helpline calls only) F: 0141 228 5912

scotland@equalityhumanrights.com

CHAPTER 10

Developing consultation skills

The previous chapters have explored the range of skills required to undertake a safe, professional consultation with a range of patient groups. The reader may be able to recognise some areas for improvement in their skills but other areas might not be so obvious. Self-evaluation is a useful tool to employ to improve skills and identify areas for further training. This final chapter offers some suggestions that the reader might find helpful for developing their consultation skills.

Self-evaluation

Self-assessment or self-evaluation is the process of critically reviewing the quality of ones own performance and provision of nursing care frequently, over time. Nurses are said to be their own toughest critics (Burns and Bulman, 2000). The process should be future orientated, as the past cannot be altered, but changes can be made to improve services or skills.

Strengths and weaknesses

Think about the main topics discussed throughout the book. Try to identify individual strengths and weaknesses. This can be the initial step to developing and/or improving consultation skills. Although an analysis of strengths, weaknesses, opportunities and threats (SWOT) conjures up a picture of academia and jargon, it is a useful tool to start the process of self evaluation. A simple example is given in Table 10.1. Everyone has elements of each category. It may be usfeul to ask a colleague to help. Identifying strengths is excellent for boosting self esteem. Identifying weaknessess is essential for improvement, while highlighting opportunities and threats enable you to consider the wider picture of developing self improvement.

Table 10.1 Personal SWOT analysis.

Strengths Good rapport with patients Conscious of body language	**Weaknesses** Too impatient and tend to interrupt Don't reflect on consultation or outcomes Do not like giving bad news
Opportunities Undertake peer review with colleagues Training to develop new skills	**Threats** Lack of time in appointments No allocated time for learning/ reflection Constant interruptions from staff

The environment

Spend some time considering whether the environment can be improved to enhance the consultation. Pretend you are the patient. What do you see when you walk into the consulting room? View this from the patient's perspective. Walk into all the rooms you use in the practice and consider the following:

- Is the room welcoming?
- Does the room appear untidy or organised?
- Does the room offer privacy?
- Is the room clean?
- Is the room temperature comfortable or is it too cold or too stuffy?
- Is the patient's chair comfortable?
- Is there a chair for a relative or companion?
- Are the patient and nurse sitting at the same eye level?
- Can the computer screen be seen? (consider confidentiality)
- Are there documents with patient details on the desk?

Refer back to Chapter 1 for guidance.

Questioning skills

The importance of using open questions to elicit information has been stressed in previous chapters. Although closed questioning may be quicker and shorten the consultation, practice using open questions. A few moments spent considering how to phrase a question will save time in the future, as these open questions will elicit more valuable information which may be vital to providing better patient care. This may require you to consciously think before you speak. Rephrase questions such as:

`How does it....?'* instead of *`Does it...'

`What can I do......'* instead of *`Do you want...?'.

`How are you feeling?'* instead of *`Do you have any pain?'

`How often do you use your brown inhaler?'* instead of, *`Do you use the brown inhaler twice a day?'

If you are conscious of using a closed question, quickly rephrase it. Remember, most patients only talk for about 30 seconds at a time, although it probably seems longer.

Listening skills

Practice your listening skills with a colleague or in a social setting. Ask someone to tell you about a particular event, such as a holiday or family event. Use active listening skills to elicit more information. For example, repeating summarised information will identify how well you `heard what was said'. Practice this skill until you feel confident that you are truly listening to the patient. Refer to Chapter 2 for techniques in active listening. In the social setting friends and family volunteer information, but how much can they say before they are interrupted? Watching other people in these situations will highlight the relevance of listening to the complete story. How do people cope with someone who speaks constantly and does not stop for breath? Watch, listen and learn.

As noted in Chapter 2, patients are usually interrupted after 15-18 seconds into their story. Discreetly time how long the patient takes to tell their story. Also note when and how often you interrupt the patient. Practice this skill until the patient is not interrupted.

Giving information

Patients may recall only a small proportion of what was said during a consultation, so it can be useful to plan sessions for chronic disease in chunks and reinforce these at subsequent visits. For example, ask an asthmatic patient to recall the advice given for self-management during an acute attack, or a diabetic to list the important issues of self-care during an illness.

- How much did they remember?

- Was it accurate?

- Had it been reinforced with literature or direction to internet resources?

Identify any areas that could be improved and spend time developing these. Patients may need to be re-educated about the details of their health care (Ward, 2008).

This activity can be transferred to management of other situations, including long term management and prevention of ulcers, ear care and travel health. Consider how to give information to people with a disability, those with poor literacy skills, and patients whose first language is not English. This might involve liaising with the multi-disciplinary team, voluntary services or local bilingual and ethnic minority (BEM) groups.

Non-verbal communication skills and body language

It can be difficult to interpret non-verbal signals but this skill can be improved by practising different types of non-verbal communication with colleagues or family. Spend ten minutes during a coffee break, or when out socially, and watch people. See how many different non-verbal signals you can identify. For example:

- Watch how people sit. Are they in an open or defensive posture?
- Is there eye contact?
- Do they fidget or play with their hair?
- Does the smile reach the eyes?
- Is someone flirting?
- Observe posture: leaning, slouching, laid back, sat up straight
- Consider head movements: nodding, shaking
- Hand movements: fidgeting, playing with hair, picking nails, drumming, waving
- Eye movements: eye contact, winking, looking down
- Facial expression: frown, smile, bored
- Body contact: shaking hands, touching
- Closeness: personal space

After observing other peoples' body language, it is also important to be conscious of your own. What vibes do you send out to others? What non-verbal messages are you sending? What is your body language saying? If you are unsure, ask a friend to be honest and point out any traits that could be improved with practice. Then practice. Ask the friend the same question three months later. Has there been improvement?

Peer review

A critical friend can be of great value, giving simple feedback during reflection (Taylor, 2006). He or she lets you talk while being non-judgemental about you as a person. The critical friend can also be a sounding board for ideas and thoughts. These could relate to improving the environment, changing the appointment system, or arranging training in consultation skills. Let the critical friend watch you undertake a consultation or procedure and then spend 15 minutes discussing their feedback. Honesty and frankness are paramount. There are always areas where improvement can be made. It is important to accept that a technique might need adaptation. That does not mean it is wrong, just that it could be improved. It might also be helpful having a colleague who is not a friend and can provide unbiased view.

Have a joint review with a colleague. Watch a colleague undertake a consultation. You might identify areas for improvement in their skills and recognise that you use the same techniques. Issues can be discussed on a one-to-one basis, or during clinical supervision. Reflect over a period of time and analyse situations from which you can gain awareness and insight.

Managing an aggressive situation

Many nurses will have experienced an aggressive situation during their training or post qualification. These include physical assault, verbal abuse, racial harassment and sexual harassment. Ask your manager to arrange a workshop for the practice staff to learn and practice basic self-defence techniques. This should include tips on identifying possible trouble and practising the methods for defusing abusive situations before they escalate (see Chapter 1). It has been reported that conflict training gives nurses the necessary skills to deal with potentially violent situations (Davis, 2007).

Think about the environment. Is there a clear escape route from the room, or can you be cornered before you can reach the door? Check that the panic button or alarm works and that help will come quickly if summoned. The nurse has a responsibility to identify health and safety issues within the environment and bring them to the attention of their manager. Ensure all safety issues are addressed.

Make a list of the unpleasant encounters you remember. What were the causes? Refer back to Chapter 1 for possible causes. What did you do? How did you feel? What have you done differently since then? This would be a useful topic for a nurses' meeting or during clinical supervision. Nurses can share their experiences and develop coping mechanisms for future encounters.

Difficult encounters

Difficult encounters differ from aggressive encounters depending on their content. These include patients who refuse to take responsibility for their own health and have a `you fix me' attitude. Consider what makes a patient `difficult' for you. This could include how you manage the patient who fails to adhere to a treatment regime for wound management. Scenario 1 demonstrates a difficult encounter for a nurse.

Role play with a colleague is an excellent way to practice technqiues to cope with these situations. This will enhance communication skills, patience and devising strategies to achieve a satisfactory outcome for all.

Supporting patients who have had bad news

The difficulties relating to both delivering bad news and supporting patients are discussed in Chapter 8. However there will be occasions when a nurse might feel she does not have the skills to do this. For example, a smear result of CIN III (severe dyskariosis) can be devastating news for any woman, but especially for one who has a family history of cervical cancer. If unable to tell the patient yourself, refer to a more experienced colleague. Be present during the consultation and watch, listen and learn. Then practice.

Labelling

It is important to consider the issue of labelling a patient. For example, is he labelled as a disease entity, someone who is always rude, or the woman with the beehive hairstyle. Labelling invites the nurse to forget the individual behind the label (Finlay, 2005). What labels do you use for patients? Are they derogatory or flattering? Have patients overheard you use these terms? Reflect on terms you use for certain patients and review your code of conduct (NMC, 2008).

Scenario 1

Mrs P has a slow healing leg ulcer. She has been attending the surgery for six weeks. The nurses have used several dressings which Mrs P removes when she gets home. The wound is now clinically infected. The nurse has taken a wound swab and the doctor has prescribed a broad-spectrum antibiotic while awaiting the result. The wound is dressed with an iodine dressing and a review booked for three days. The wound is still erythematous, malodorous and has large exudates. Tissue paper is adhered to the wound.

Nurse: "Hello, Mrs P. How are you feeling today?"

Mrs P "That dressing hurt, so I took it off yesterday."

Nurse: "The wound still looks sore. Are you taking the tablets that the doctor prescribed?"

Mrs P: "No. I read the side effects and decided not to take them."

The reader can probably relate this scenario to many encounters. How did you manage it?

Options:
1. Spend more time explaining the benefits of the antibiotics and reassuring Mrs P that the side effects are short lived.
2. Change the antibiotic.
3. Apply a simple dressing to the wound.
4. Consider doppler and four layer bandaging to stop Mrs Peters interfering with the wound.
5. Refer to a wound care specialist.
6. All of the above.

Communicating with people who are deaf or hard of hearing

As there are an estimated 9 million deaf and hard of hearing adults in the UK (Royal National Institute for Deaf People, 2009), many patients and/or relatives who attend general practice have some level of hearing loss. It is difficult to consult effectively without two-way communication. There are many ways to manage this consultation. Practice the following exercise with a colleague. Sit facing each other. Use headphones to block out noise and try to lip read your colleague's speech. This can heighten awareness of the need to speak slowly and not exaggerate lip movements. Repeat this with your colleague reading your lips. This will identify the clarity of your speech. Practice until you feel confident to lip-read.

Cultural diversity

The United Kingdom is a culturally diverse country. Think of a consultation with a patient who was raised in a different culture and where you felt frustrated at not being able to offer optimum care. What made the consultation frustrating? Issues could include:

• Lack of time for translation
• No interpreter
• Not understanding health beliefs and cultural norms

Do you know how many different BME groups are registered with the practice? This information is available from the census data. Consider devising a practice folder with information about each group, including health beliefs. It could be useful to involve local minority groups, including gypsy travellers and asylum seekers, in the design and delivery of any cultural training. Ask the Primary Care Trust to organise cultural awareness workshops if not already in operation. A small directory could include useful contacts for websites, addresses and telephone numbers detailing services for different minority groups.

Videotaping

Videotaped consultations, with patient consent, are useful learning exercises in review the consultation structure, the use of body language and communication skills (Brant, 2007). This model is used in training practices, where doctors are videotaped undertaking a consultation. The following guides for videotaping patients has been adapted from Patient UK (2007) for practice nurses.

Consent

The patient's consent for this consultation should be gained prior to them entering the consultation room. Offer the patient a consent form that includes a brief explanation of what is involved, advising who will view the recording, and if they wish to change their mind the camera will be switched off and that section erased. It is essential to stress the confidentiality aspect of the recording. A nurse who has a good rapport with her patients and explains the rationale behind videotaping the consultation should have little difficulty gaining consent from a number of patients for this method of self-improvement.

Process

The camera should be set up to discreetly capture the patient's face and expressions and preferably include the nurse too. The tape is then watched with a colleague or trainer. This offers the opportunity for discussion and reflection. The trainee and trainer can identify areas for improvement. Although nurses might be uncomfortable being videotaped, this model offers an ideal opportunity for all nurses to improve their consultation skills as everyone has something to improve upon.

Reflection

After watching the tape, the nurse states what he or she thought went well, before moving onto aspects that might have been done better. The colleague or trainer then offers positive comments before highlighting areas for improvement.

Data protection

Storage of any digital records must be kept secure and agreement made on the lifespan for keeping recordings. Records could be subject to inappropriate use if mislaid or lost.

Although a time consuming process, videotaping of developing consultation skills is worth the effort. It incorporates all the aspects of communication given and received, allows assessment of body language and listening skills and enables nurses to see directly how they perform in a practical situation.

Patient feedback

Obtain feedback from the patient on how they felt during the consultation. This could be an anonymous questionnaire or verbal feedback. Comments could relate to any aspect of the consultation, including time management, environment, questioning and listening skills. Nurses should be able to accept criticism positively and appreciate the opportunity to make changes to consultations.

Self-directed study

Although time is often a perceived barrier to learning there are always opportunities to read articles and books. This might be reading one article while in the bath, reading a journal when travelling by train, or by dipping into a textbook when time permits. A GP training practice library should have copies of consultation skill books that can be borrowed, or read on the premises. This is an excellent use of professional learning time and clinical supervision. There is a wealth of information available in the Royal College of Nursing and nursing libraries to supplement the previous chapters.

Reflective practice

Clinical supervision is one forum for exploring the emotional problems relating to incidents, including delivering or sharing bad news. Reflection on past experiences and discussion with colleagues offers nurses the opportunity to increase their self awareness and meet individual professional needs, leading in turn to improved patient care (Edwards, 2008).

E-mail consultations

Discuss the pros and cons of e-mail consultations with colleagues. Is there a place for this in practice? Do other practices use this method for follow up consultations or patient advice? Explore the legal aspects, develop a protocol, trial a pilot and ask for feedback from patients. Although not suitable for all consultations, it has the potential to reduce lost messages, enables replying directly to patient queries, and is an alternative for patients who are hard of hearing or have difficulty accessing the surgery.

Summary

Practice nurses consult in every patient intervention, whether formally or passing the time of day in the waiting room. They are alert to the patient's body language and physical symptoms. The maxim to follow is surely "Do as I would be done by", and treat all patients and their relatives, regardless of sexuality, disability or race, in the manner you wish for yourself, your family and your friends. Bear this is mind when you next welcome a patient into the consulting room, gain a history and undertake any physical intervention. Consider privacy, dignity, respect and confidentiality. Listen. Let the patient speak.

The best feeling in the world is when a patient says;

"Thank you. You're the only person who has really listened to me".

Brant C (2007) The nurse will see you. *Nursing Standard.* **22**(13): 62-3

Burns S & Bulman C (2000) *Reflective Practice in Nursing. The Growth of the Reflective Practitioner.* 2nd Ed. Oxford, Blackwell Science Ltd. Davis C (2007) Keeping the peace. *Nursing Standard.* **22**(12): 18-9

David C (2007) keeping the peace. *Nursing Standard* **229** (12): 18-9

Edwards M (2008) *The Informed Practice Nurse* 2nd Ed. Chichester, Wiley Finlay L (2005) Difficult encounters. *Nursing Management.* **12**(1): 31-5

Finlay L (2005) Difficult encounters. *Nursing Management* **12** (1): 31-5

Nursing and Midwifery Council (2008) *The Code. Standards of conduct, performance and ethics for nurses and midwives.* London, NMC

Patient UK (2007) *Consultation Analysis.* www.patient.co.uk accessed 11/10/2008

Royal National Institute for Deaf people (2009) Statistics. www.rnid.org.uk <http://www.rnid.org.uk> accessed 8/11/2009

Taylor BJ (2006) *Reflective Practice. A Guide for Nurses and Midwives.* 2nd Ed. Maidenhead, Open University Press

Ward P (2008) Why do people with diabetes fall off the rails? T*he British Journal of Primary Care Nursing.* **5**(5): 251-3

Index